Back Talk

Other Books by Eric Nicol

Sense and Nonsense
The Roving I
Twice Over Lightly
Shall We Join the Ladies?
Girdle Me a Globe
An Uninhibited History of Canada (with Peter Whalley)
In Darkest Domestica
Say, Uncle (with Peter Whalley)
A Herd of Yaks (with Peter Whalley)
Russia, Anyone? (with Peter Whalley)
Space Age, Go Home!
100 Years of What? (with Peter Whalley)
A Scar Is Born
Don't Move!
Vancouver
The Best of Eric Nicol
Letters to My Son
There's a Lot of It Going Around
Still a Nicol
One Man's Media
Canada Cancelled – Because of Lack of Interest
The Joy of Hockey (with Dave More)
The Joy of Football (with Dave More)
Golf – The Agony & the Ecstasy (with Dave More)
Canadide
How To . . . (with Graham Pilsworth)
Tennis – It Serves You Right (with Dave More)
The U.S. or Us (with Dave More)
Dickens of the Mounted

Back Talk

A Book for Bad-Back Sufferers

and Those Who L̶o̶v̶e̶ ᴘᴜᴛ ᴜᴘ ᴡɪᴛʜ Them

Eric Nicol

Illustrated by Graham Pilsworth

⟦A DOUGLAS GIBSON BOOK⟧

M&S

This is a book of humour. None of the characters portrayed here are real, nor are their names, and none of the "medical" opinions represent anything other than the opinion of the author, a layman (sitting or standing is hard for him).

Canadian Cataloguing in Publication Data
Nicol, Eric, 1919–
  Back talk : a book for bad-back sufferers and those who love (put up with) them

ISBN 0–7710–6809–3 `

1. Backache – Humor.   I. Pilsworth, Graham, 1944–   .
II. Title.

PS8527.I46B32 1992   C617.5'64'00207   C92–094586–4
PR9199.3.N42B32 1992

Printed and bound in Canada
The paper used in this book is acid-free

A Douglas Gibson Book

McClelland & Stewart Inc.
The Canadian Publishers
481 University Avenue
Toronto, Ontario
M5G 2E9

Printed and bound in Canada by Best Gagné Book Manufacturers

Contents

Dedicated . . .

to all those back-pain victims
who have suffered in silence . . .
and to the other 99% of us
who scream like banshees

But those behind cried "Forward!"
And those before cried "Back!"

– Lord Macaulay, *Lays of Ancient Rome*, "Horatius"

Pre-op

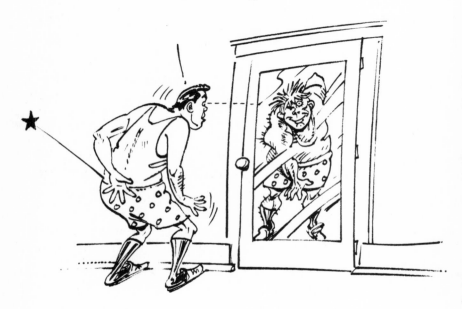

You have a bad back. Nearly all of us (75-90 per cent) at some point in our lives claim to have a bad back. (Interestingly, even though the front is easier to see, hardly anyone ever complains of having a bad front.) Yet such is the mystique of the bad back that back pain is responsible for more lost work time in North America than any other mentionable excuse, except the flu bug. Compensation benefits run to as much as $70 billion a year, which is why workers' compensation boards wince just picking up the tab.

Despite this mass production of bad backs, dorsal dolour is the prestigious ailment of the nineties. The bad back has taken over from old favourites like gout and the vapours as today's most respectable reason for going to the doctor. Yet anyone can afford the conditions for a bad back. White-collar workers, blue-collar workers, *no*-collar workers (among whom I am proud to be numbered) – regardless of class, age, sex, or religion – we can all attribute our bad back to something admirable: *hard work*. Whether in the farm field or on the tennis court, in the executive swivel chair or in kitchen, warehouse, or whorehouse, our bad back has been hard earned. That's more than can be said for mumps.

We bad-backers even tend to look down on people with heart problems – compassionately, mind you – since the chances are that they have smoked tobacco, gorged on polysaturated fats, stressed themselves out, locked themselves in, and exercised only at gunpoint. In contrast, Back People have no shame. We bow to no one. Not without help. The worst that a critic can say of us is that we have loved not wisely but too well, in positions that seemed like fun at the time but contributed to a herniated disc.

Far from being an unmitigated handicap, the bad back may actually enhance the charisma of authority. President John F. Kennedy gained stature for conducting vigorous campaigns, both in and out of America's bedrooms, despite his volatile vertebrae. He successfully converted the seat of power to a rocking-chair. His bad back had mass appeal, yet was more stylish than "the king's disease" (epilepsy) with which Julius Caesar awed the populace but rarely got a laugh. And as an emblem of leadership, Napoleon's hemorrhoids were clearly a non-starter.

In Canadian politics, former Liberal party leader John Turner won the nation's admiration, though not enough votes, when he fought the '89 election despite being on the limp from a fractious back. He proved that the bad back is *the* democratic affliction, after the House of Commons. Unlike Richard III – who with Quasimodo gave having a bad back a bad name for centuries – Turner was never driven to putting someone in the Peace Tower.

Ultimate endorsement of the bad back: Wayne Gretzky – with Mario Lemieux not far behind.

Because having a bad back is chic without being frivolous, many people hate to give it up. They will do anything for their bad back except actually cure it. They resort to ice-packs, heat-packs, back-packs (masochists), bags of frozen peas, belts, braces, corsets, special shoes, special insoles worn with special socks, back-rests, foot-rests, neck-rests, the defence rests, special pillows, special chairs, special beds made specially in Sweden of special wood and equipped with airbags, special mattresses, special boards under the special mattresses, and, presumably, special bags of frozen peas for princesses with bad backs.

None of these items actually *cure* the bad back. But they may help you. And they certainly make grand topics of conversation, and keep the economy moving. Many economists now look to housing starts, car sales, and the development of new bad-back devices as the major indicators of health in the modern economy.

Also, armies of people are involved in tending bad backs, besides doctors, nurses, and vets. Bad backs provide gainful employment to myriad chiropractors, naturopaths, acupuncturists, yoga or shiatsu or tai-chi gurus, physiotherapists, and Yellow Pages masseuses who let their fingers do the walking. It has been estimated that while 10 per cent of the adult population is suffering from a back attack at any given moment, another 10 per cent is gainfully employed in trying to fix them.

To try to relieve the sciatic pain in *my* legs, I bought one of those inversion contraptions that hang you upside-down by the ankles, the purpose being to fool the vertebrae into thinking that you have swung back into the trees, as nature intended. As every bad-backer knows, his or her trouble began when a fool male baboon stood on his hind legs in order to get a better look at a female flashing her pink behind. If our ancestors had been smart enough to remain on all fours, the pressure on our spine would be relieved, though it might be harder to get a good table at the Ritz.

I used my inverter – which cost about two hundred bucks, but held out hopes of a blissful back – only once. Even though my wife, who is an RN and fully qualified to supervise medical equipment, monitored my gradual reversal, I was still several degrees short of perpendicular when I cracked, yelling "Yes! I abjure heresy! God bless King Ferdinand and the Pope!" My wife righted me before I could inform on *her*.

Thereafter I used the inverter only to frighten small children who came to visit us. After I had barked my shin on its unforgiving steel frame for the umpteenth time, I called in a rubbish removal outfit and persuaded the crew to take it away free. "You'll find," I told them, "that it's a wonderful ice-breaker for parties. Especially mixed parties."

However, some bad-backers swear by their inverters. And the apparatus does seem somewhat safer than gravity boots. A friend of mine strapped a pair on his feet and proceeded to hang from his kitchen door frame. It did his back the world of good until the door frame collapsed under the weight. He is scheduled for cervical surgery, his neck now being too short for his shirt collars.

The reason why people find such a plenitude of ways to placate their bad back is that there are *good* bad backs and *bad* bad backs. A good bad back is one that "goes out" at the right moment, like an hour before you are due to go to your brother-in-law's funeral. Conversely, when *you* want to go out, your good bad back stays *in* – for that trip to Vegas, say, or just a quiet stroll to the pub. I had a good bad back for about ten years, before it became a liability. I played tennis and badminton as strenuously as before my back went bad, but if I lost the game I left the court clutching my lumbar region. To effectively destroy the satisfaction of other club members in beating me, I also made a show of placing my cane in my locker before start of play. The only member who could really enjoy kicking my butt was a guy who had had a triple bypass. I tried to avoid playing against him. Some people *flaunt* their handicap.

Other useful exercises in bad–backmanship for the games player:

• After doing the usual stretching exercises, at length, before playing a game, lie down on your stomach and ask your opponent to walk on your back. Explain that this is necessary to prevent your spinal cord from kinking.

• Wear a medical belt *above* your sports clothes. Do not refer to it. If asked by your opponent, explain that your back can go into spasm at any point, and you're so tired of being rushed into Emergency that you take every precaution.

• Shyly ask your opponent if he or she would mind picking up the ball every time, since stooping is so hard for you. In tennis this ploy alone is a match–winner. In golf this *can* be extended to asking your opponent to tee up for you.

• Leave one shoelace loosely tied. When it comes undone, ask your opponent if he or she would mind tying it up. At this point the game is as good as won. You have become a charge to be looked after, not an opponent to be beaten. However . . .

• If you are somehow at the point of losing, forget your rule about stooping, then freeze while bending over to retrieve your ball. Remain at ninety degrees to the floor (court, grass, etc.), till carried or driven to Emergency.

But what happens when you run out of ploys? When all the crows come home to roost, right on your sciatic nerve? When, dammit, you have to *do* something about that bad back?

Such is the matter of this slim volume. (Kept slim, of course, to avoid a problem with the book's spine, which is guaranteed to stay glued longer than the author's.) The chapters that follow are intended to focus the fears of the candidate for back surgery, and provide a bit of ether-scented nostalgia for the veteran of that somewhat harrowing interlude . . . keeping in mind that back trauma is rarely aggravated by smiling.

In my own case, far from anticipating back surgery, for years I didn't even know that it was my back that was responsible for the frightful pain in my leg and numbness in the foot. I attributed my discomfort to an unknown and probably unspeakable condition, resulting from sexual excesses, cheap sneakers, or some other cause of which I had every reason to feel ashamed. Only when *in extremis* did I go to a doctor and confess that God was punishing me for wearing snug underwear.

The doctor cut me short. He didn't want to hear my carefully rehearsed and somewhat expurgated account of the self-abuse of my youth. Instead he sent me for X-rays, which he subsequently reported to reveal that my lower spine was turning to pea gravel.

"Osteoarthritis," he said matter-of-factly. "The disc is just worn out. Happens to nearly everybody when they grow old."

It had never occurred to me that I might grow old. I should perhaps have suspected something when my hair turned grey and the numbers in the telephone book mysteriously started to shrink. But like anyone else I associated aging with other people, those unfortunate enough to be physically affected by the passage of time. (On reflection, I believe that the possibility of growing old should be taught in school, along with sex education, since both sex and aging are occurrences that can happen to *anybody*.)

"Rest," the doctor told me, "is the best cure for a condition like yours. Just learn to take it easy."

I was so grateful for this over-the-counter prescription that I immediately resumed playing racquet games, adding jogging as another activity that I could rest after, too late. But it still hurt, just to play backgammon.

A few years and another doctor later, my *left* leg started humming the refrain from everything. I had begun to walk and stand at a canted angle. The full-length mirror told me that I was taking on a growing resemblance to the Hunchback of Notre Dame (the Charles Laughton version). I mentioned the problem to Dr. Fine during a routine examination. To my dismay he paid attention to what I was mumbling. I had clearly chosen the wrong doctor. My previous doctor had been an older man, slightly deaf, prepared to die and let die. Dr. Fine, in contrast, is a young, tall, handsome athlete who has the sickening idea that everyone, regardless of age, has a right to enjoy the misery of playing thirty-six holes of golf.

"I *hate* golf," I told him truthfully, as he made a note on my file. "I don't miss it a bit. All I want is to have enough play in my shaft to let me pick up a quarter from the sidewalk without my vertebrae playing the castanet concerto."

"You told me you're a frustrated jock." (That damn file – I have to figure a way to burn it.) "You're in pretty good shape for your age. If you don't stay active you'll become a couch potato."

The ugly part of his comment was that it was true. All of it. I *had* blabbed to him that I depended on ping-pong to purge the aggression that otherwise makes my face break out. And I *was* already well on my way to becoming a sofa spud, a chaise-longue legume, with eyes sprouting in the germinal glow of the schlock box. But before I could tell Dr. Fine that I was looking forward to becoming a veggie, he scribbled a name on his notepad. "I'm going to give you a referral, to Dr. Goodbody. He's one of the best."

"Best *what*?"

"Neurosurgeons. If I were having back surgery, he'd be my man."

The word "surgery" sent a shiver up my spine – a farewell appearance? I had already talked to a lot of people about back surgery. None of them had had back surgery themselves, but he or she knew someone who had had it and was now playing basketball – in a wheel-chair. Next to the collected works of Stephen King, no horror stories are more popular than those listed under the general title How Freddy Got Filleted.

The only previous surgery I'd had in my life was the stitching together of an Achilles' tendon ruptured when I tried to make a Rod Laver rush to the net. I had done so without giving due consideration to the fact that, after fifty, the sinews in a man's hams can dry out to the consistency of cheesesticks. After *sixty*, it's a lucky tennis player who hears a string pop and it's in his racquet.

But surgical repair of one's extremities involves a much lower anxiety factor than that of the stack of discs that makes the torso our favourite jukebox. Per-haps noticing the twitch of my wattles, Dr. Fine added:

"You can always cancel the appointment if you change your mind."

I liked the sound of that. Indeed, I needed it. I have always been in such awe of the doctor in the white coat that it would never occur to me to change my mind if it might inconvenience him. Or her. But especially him. I have had little experience with being intimidated by a woman doctor. Since *any* woman makes me feel inadequate, even when I'm fully dressed, I have avoided being treated by a female physician. The only time I found myself confronted by one – she was subbing for my regular doctor – I hastily relocated my abdominal cramps to above the belt. This nonplussed the lady MD, but I was damned if I was going to drop my drawers in front of a woman without knowing more about what amused her. Result: she diagnosed as a possible kidney stone what proved to be wind in the southern hemisphere.

"Okay," I told Dr. Fine. "I'll make an appointment with Dr. Goodbody that I can cancel at very short notice – right?"

"No problem," smiled Dr. Fine. Did he know something I didn't?

1

The Qualm Before the Storm

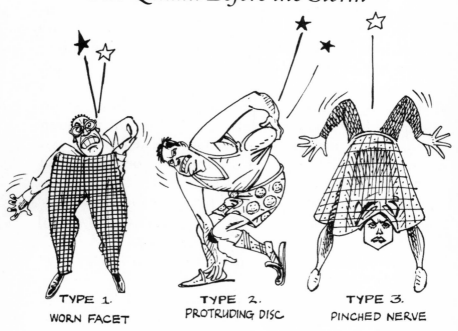

TYPE 1.
WORN FACET

TYPE 2.
PROTRUDING DISC

TYPE 3.
PINCHED NERVE

The main problem with repeated cancellation of the medical appointment as a method of treating a bad back is that the relief from pain tends to be short-lived. Your back feels better till you hang up the phone. Then the sciatic or dorsal anguish returns fiercer than ever, and you have to make another appointment with the doctor's secretary, who may show signs of concluding that in your resolve you fall somewhere short of Winston Churchill.

I rationalized my procrastination as prudence, a period for sound, personal research into bad backs, so that I could make an informed judgment whether to go for the surgery or stay with what doctors like to call conservative measures, such as proper posture, special exercises, and hanging a picture of Brian Mulroney above my bed.

I was particularly impressed by the bad-back literature recommendation of the bar-rail, on which to rest one foot when obliged to stand for any length of time.

"What I need," I told my wife, "is a *portable* bar-rail, a bar-rail I can take to cocktail parties, church weddings, supermarket checkouts . . ."

"Have the operation," said my wife. Women don't understand the role of high tech in back therapy.

More comforting were the back-doctor books, especially those chapters that urged the bad-backer to avoid surgery if possible, by adopting proper living habits. Carrying the bride across the threshold is asking for trouble, I noted, and can be almost as damaging if the couple are not married. Lift with the legs, not the

back, instructed the manuals. I observed this rule with
a religiousness bordering on fanaticism, yet was surprised to find how many toting situations do not lend
themselves to the leg lift. Unloading the trunk of the
car, for instance. Unless you bring the groceries home
on a dog sled, you will perforce bend into the vehicle,
and if your back locks up you may have to be hoisted
clear by a CAA man.

Other no-nos: never try to lift a heavy roast out of
the oven. You may be found by loved ones, your face
baked to a turn. Cook nothing heavier than bacon.

At the airport, watch the baggage carousel but make
no attempt to retrieve your bag from it. Just let it go
round and round till an old lady takes it off by mistake,
then wrestle it away from her. Chiropractors buy
Mercedes on the strength of the number of patients
brought to them directly from the airport. Some have a
deal with airport taxi drivers.

Equally disillusioning are the back-book chapters
describing the different grades of back problem. The
most common, almost vulgar, type is referred to when
your doctor tells you, "You have a cute back pain." If
you reply, "Thanks, doc, yours is kinda neat too," you
have misheard. What your doctor is trying to tell you is
that you have pranged a tendon, muscle, ligament,
cartilage, or other rigging on the old mainmast. This is
called "a soft-tissue injury," and can happen to young
people as well as to us older folk who have put in a
lifetime cultivating our hardware injury to the discs
and mortar. We elders tend to sneer at software back
pain, since the remedy for it is usually rest and painkil-
lers – kid stuff. Oh, yes, we know that it hurts, son or
daughter, when your back goes into spasm, but you
likely won't be told to have surgery, and therein lies the

tail-bone. Mind you, if you persist well into your fifties in your bad habits of posture, dancing the twist or the lambada while weighing three hundred pounds, you too may graduate to our elite class: God's cloven people.

This class is often divided into Type One (the Worn Facet), Type Two (the Protruding Disc), and Type Three (the Pinched Nerve). Types One and Two are the most common and the easiest to live with, so long as you find the right balance between martyrdom and Aspirin. Type Three can eventually result in nerve damage, loss of muscle strength, and a foot that flaps like a scuba diver's flipper.

I tried the do-it-yourself tests in hopes of establishing that I was only a Type One, or better yet a Type One-third. The results being inconclusive, I decided that I must be the extremely rare Type Four (Type One plus Type Three, or Compact Disc With Long Play). The more reading I did, the stronger grew the suspicion that my back problem was incurable, inoperable, and indecent. Worst of all, sitting reading all the back books aggravated the pain in my legs, though I sat with my legs properly raised on a pouffe and with prescribed glasses.

Hence my taking the heroic measure of making an appointment with Dr. Goodbody and keeping it. A medical breakthrough. The walk from the parking-lot to his office – a matter of a couple of blocks – would have been the perfect time for the numbing pain down my legs to go into remission. My mind was eminently receptive to any physical sign, however slight, that would cast doubt on the need to actually enter the surgeon's office. It didn't have to be something as spectacular as a sudden urge to hurdle hedges. *Any* small mercy would be gratefully received – a reduced need to wince at each step . . . a bit more Fred Astaire in the way I was dragging my left foot . . .

No joy. When I limped into the doctor's office, my back was stating, in italics, that I was in the right place, about two years late.

"The doctor will be with you shortly," smiled his secretary. "If you care to take a seat in the waiting-room."

The doctor's waiting-room. The absolutely last chance for the patient to chicken out. An even better chance to study the other patients trying to act cool as they flip through magazines held upside down. It was in one of these I once read that some doctors have installed Waiting-Room TV, as an incentive for the patient to remain till his or her name is called. Pediatricians offer shows like "Baby's First Visit to the Doctor." Dentists, I gather, run some pretty dramatic features on flossing. And I can see the value of videos on breast self-examination, if I could find an excuse for being in the clinic. But in *this* doctor's waiting-room I had to settle for the inevitable year-old copy of *The Reader's Digest*, in which the main article was entitled something like "Unnecessary Surgery – The New Plague."

Dr. Goodbody fetched me forth personally. A tall, slim, youngish man, he watched my gait as I walked beside him into his office. Jeez, he was estimating the odds before I even got out of the paddock. I put as much verve as I could into sitting down, while he sat behind his desk and opened his notebook. In his amateur concert-party comedy act, my father used to get laughs with the line "She went into the doctor's office and he took down her particulars." Patter familias. I thought it was pretty funny, too, till my own particulars were taken down, again and again. Maybe it's the kind of sketch that needs a live studio audience.

I was mentally prepared for the tests the doctor put me through. I had done my homework and cut my toenails. When he took me into his examining-room and told me to walk on my heels, I was ready. I not only walked on them, I made it look as though this were my preferred method of ambulation. I gave a new dimension to ankling, reminiscent of the Paris postmen's walking race.

"Mm." Dr. Goodbody didn't seem as impressed as I'd hoped by this vigorous demonstration that the nerve damage in my legs was not dire enough to prevent me from dancing *sur les points*, though a career as another Nureyev was iffy. "Sit on the table, please."

I vaulted nimbly, almost, onto the examining-table, alert to what would come next: the old reflex test. A veteran of watching the rubber hammer strike me below the knee, with no response whatever from the wretched nerve, I was primed to swing my foot at the precise moment of impact. The timing has to be exquisite for this place-kick to be convincing. Jerk your lower limb too soon, before the hammer has hit the knee, and you boot your credibility.

"Hey!" I exclaimed. "I guess the nerve isn't dead after all. Maybe I'm wasting your time, doctor – "

"Close your eyes. Tell me if you feel these pricks."

Aha! The human pincushion bit. I've submitted to it so often I'm an honorary member of the Calcutta Fakirs Association. The drill is that the doctor impales your toes and the soles of your feet on a pin, moving up the outside of your calves and creating an inkless tattoo that spells I LOVE LULU.

This test was as close as I ever got to acupuncture as a remedy for my back problem. Having additional pins and needles in my feet was just painting the lily, in my view. I had given acupuncture a pretty good trial every time I darned my socks. But, to be fair, I have friends who swear by it. In any case, this pin test posed unusual challenges to my alertness.

"Yes, yes, I felt that," I told the doctor. "And that . . . and that . . . "

"I haven't started yet."

"No? My big toe must have sensed your approach. It's a kind of sonar my feet have, ha, ha. Ah, well, I do flatter myself that my sensory perception is better than average. Let me know when you start pricking."

"I've finished. Lie on your back, please."

I was confident about lying on my back. It is one of my more accessible positions, more feasible even than lying on my stomach. And I was prepared for the doctor's trying to push my legs apart while I strove to keep them together – the way Mother taught me a good girl should. Also, I had good muscle tone in my thighs, thanks to years of recreational biking and weeding. My wife has commended my glutes. My socks stay up, though my calves are more dependent than formerly on the grip of the varicose veins.

Thus I was able to give a good account of myself in the hand-to-ham combat with the good doctor. Eat your heart out, Gorgeous Ladies of Wrestling!

Having completed the descent from the examining-table, I stood while the doctor checked my vital signs: SLOW . . . PREPARE TO STOP . . . DEAD END . . . This routine procedure always alarms me because – am I alone in this? – I have never been able to find my pulse, and I fear that one day the doctor won't either. Embarrassment for all concerned. Similarly, when the doctor takes my blood pressure, and has to squeeze that black bulb repeatedly because the air is escaping through my navel, I half expect him to announce that my blood is under no pressure at all. Which would explain why I have never had my photo in the *National Enquirer*.

"Take a deep breath."

I knew why he needed to confirm that I was a lung breather. When I am being wheeled into the operating-room is no time for the anesthetist to discover that I respire through gills. But I don't really like having to take deep breaths, because normally I avoid inhaling. The air is so polluted in the city that I try to confine my breathing to exhaling. Consequently, when I *do* take a deep breath, on doctor's orders, the unaccustomed rush of oxygen into my lungs makes me light-headed and giddy.

"Tee-hee," I tittered. "Look, doc – my chest doesn't expand, but my nipples inflate."

"Take another deep breath."

Wow! Two deep breaths in one day! I hope this isn't addictive. . . .

"Okay, you can get dressed now." From the way the doctor was frowning at his notes, I surmised that I had flunked as a candidate for major back surgery. I would just have to live with the pain, becoming progressively more bent over till I looked like one of those little old men of the Orient who beetle along with their nose about a foot from the ground.

On the plus side, all the back books agreed that as a person grows *really* old the pain subsides, the body somehow attaining the state of inertia for which I have a natural aptitude. Why kid myself that I have the same prospects as young folk – football players, free-style skiers, ballet dancers – who would have to wait years for their backs to atrophy?

Having been rejected for surgery, I could comfortably assume the noble stance of letting youth have prior claim to our very busy medical services. I could hear myself telling people, as I leaned gallantly on my cane: "Yes, the pain *is* excruciating, but who am I to occupy a hospital bed when little Timmy is waiting on his crutches?"

This pleasant reverie was shattered by Dr. Goodbody's completing his notes with: "Well, you certainly seem fit enough for the surgery."

"I *am*?" My heart sank, too late to affect my cardiac rating. How could my body do this to me? Screw little Timmy, this is *my* future we're talking about.

Was this all the thanks I got for abstaining from tobacco, hard liquor, promiscuous sex, pay TV? Betrayal! One chance for my physical condition to make a good impression, and it has to be on this surgeon, not on the Dallas Cowboys cheer-leaders. I said hoarsely: "You think I would survive the operation, even though I have a history of hay fever?"

"I'd say your chances are excellent. Occasionally the patient has a problem because he or she is obese, but you should be okay."

Too late, I saw that I should have waddled into his office with a mag spare tire. Now it was too late to tell him that I was lean only because I had just emerged from hibernation, it being July. Dr. Goodbody was already saying, "I'd like you to have a myelogram before the surgery. You may arrange it with my secretary."

The interview was over. I still had a shopping-list of questions I wanted to ask him, such as:

• Was the operation's success rate affected by the patient's never having been baptized?

• Since the operating-rooms of the hospital are in a prime earthquake zone, overdue for "the Big One," what is the procedure in case the building collapses just as I am being cleaved?

• Was he, my surgeon, enjoying a happy home life? No serious problems with cabbage worm? Children? Booze? His broker? Gambling debts?

But I forbore. There is such a thing as showing *too* much concern about surviving an operation. No one admires a person who seems to overvalue his continued existence. More estimable is he or she who displays a cavalier disregard for risk, in the spirit of Churchill, who on various battle fronts made a point of standing in exposed positions so that later he could write: "There is nothing more exhilarating than being shot at, without effect."

However, before I left his office, I asked Dr. Goodbody to write down the name for the surgery he proposed: *a decompressive laminectomy*. That struck me agog. In sheer volume of syllables alone, it outclassed a butt lift. It sounded more exotic than the conventional discotomy – the relatively prosaic removal of part of a disc – without the terrifying connotation of the spinal fusion, in which the vertebrae are welded together with strips of bone taken from the rear of the pelvis – a hell of a way for your back to make an ass of itself.

Let the decompressive chips fall where they may!

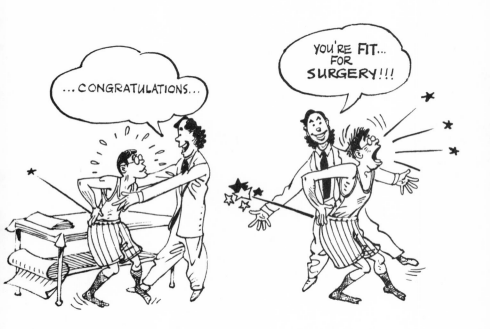

2

X-rated – Frequent Scenes of Horror

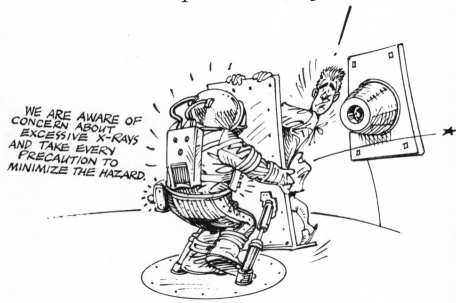

A myelogram. The Ingmar Bergman of X-rays. The one X-ray that causes even the most hardened doctor, the one who can stand any amount of your pain, to cough delicately "Not – ahem – a very pleasant procedure."

Like all truly dedicated bad-back sufferers, I had already had so many X-rays of my spine I was starting to fear that they would have to bury me in a concrete box. Deep in the desert of New Mexico. With the first of these back X-rays, I was afraid that the radiologist would report that I was not a vertebrate. The sort of medical discovery that is hard to keep out of the journals: a mature male with a valid driver's licence has been found to be a highly evolved type of sponge. Eventually the media pick up a story like that, and then I see it in the eyes of those around me: there goes the neighbourhood.

Having escaped the first X-ray without international exposure, I switched my anxiety to how much is too much. I developed the following guide, to tell whether the diagnosis of your back problem has involved too many X-rays:

- All the hair falls off your cat.
- Your spouse puts on a lead apron before sex. Or during.
- The wallet you carry in your back pocket mutates into something that snaps at your hand.
- Your house glows in the dark. Neighbours call it "Three Mile Island."
- There's no need to buy a microwave – the food cooks in your mouth.

Every Radiology guest room I've been ushered into has a sign on the wall that says something like this: WE ARE AWARE OF CONCERN ABOUT EXCESSIVE X-RAYS AND TAKE EVERY PRECAUTION TO MINIMIZE THE HAZARD.

That's why there is no one in the room except you.

The X-ray technician – usually a woman – makes an appearance as brief as possible. You are not given time enough to establish a real relationship. Having made sure that you are squarely on the griddle, she disappears into a bunker, from which she controls the machine. Her instructions – conveyed by intercom – consist mostly of "Hold your breath." No problem. I have been holding my breath since I walked in from the parking-lot. What's another three seconds? Or three minutes? If I'm scared enough, I can hold my breath indefinitely. I have had so much experience in Radiology, I could make it as a Japanese pearl-diver, once I'd brushed up on the swimming part of it.

From time to time the technician returns to the death chamber to flip you, to make sure that you are done on both sides. I have been in the rotisserie many times, being X-rayed by the old-fashioned machine that uses plates like the ones the photographer used to take pictures of your great-great-grandfather. The X-rays are pretty grainy and usually indicate that your spine has a handlebar moustache.

Not that I ever saw *my* X-rays. That's one of the odd things about this type of photography: everyone gets to see the pictures except the subject. He or she has no opportunity to laugh or cry, looking at the pictures, or to order prints to include with Christmas cards.

The reason given for this is of course that only the radiologist can "read" your X-rays. It would take too long for him to take you on his knee and read them to you ("See Disc. See Disc slip. . . ."). Instead, the radiologist reports only to your doctor. Your doctor won't let you see the pictures either. He doesn't have them. They have already been locked in a vault somewhere, a repository where all the old X-rays are stacked, and anyone who opens the tomb becomes subject to the curse (terminal dandruff). If you want to know what your X-rays looked like, you have to have more X-rays.

If I were to hazard a guess as to what eventually becomes of the millions of X-rays taken every year, it would be that they are recycled as placemats in Hell.

But the elementary X-rays of my back with ordinary radiology equipment did not alarm me as much as what I read in the back books about that Hitler of invasive probes: the myelogram. The thought of having a dye needled into my spinal fluid put the wind straight up my drawers. I don't even dye my *hair*. I have only one life to live: let me live it as a blond . . . brunette . . . redhead – anything but a peroxide scut. I doubted that having tinted vertebrae would heighten my appeal on the beach, even if I could choose my own shade.

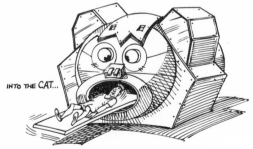

INTO THE CAT...

I therefore wangled from my personal physician a referral for a CAT scan. I liked everything I had read about the CAT scan. Even its full name – Computerized

Axial Tomography – resonated with *le dernier cri*. On
TV I had seen patients being gently fed into the scanner. They looked relaxed and happy. All they had to do
was lie there while the immense and trustworthy
machine slowly revolved around them. I am predis-
posed towards anything that revolves around me, the
family having disappointed me in this respect. More-
over, the scanner costs a million dollars, plus another
half-million a year to operate. I'm worth it. I feel sorry
for bad-backers who live in rural areas and lack access
to a large hospital that can afford the scanner, but there
has to be *some* compensation for suffering smog and
city traffic.

As I understood it, the CAT scan shows more-detailed
views of the spine than regular X-rays, slicing the
offending vertebrae into thin sections and teaching
them a good lesson. The magically reassembled pix
facilitate the doctor's scrutiny so that he may – just may
– discover that surgery is not needed after all, that your
back will be right as rain if you eat more often at Greek
restaurants and watch how the belly dancer stays supple.

So it was with a positive attitude that I accepted the
blue gown from the clerk at the reception desk of the
Radiology Department.

"Just leave your clothes in the locker," she instructed
me, "but keep your wallet." All hospitals are solicitous
about the welfare of your wallet or purse. You may lose
any other appendage without upsetting the institution
("Really? The *left* leg? Oh jeez."), but it takes every
precaution against premature separation of body and
sous.

Unfortunately, the standard hospital gown does not
have a pocket. This means that the patient, when

moving from changing cubicle to the theatre of operation (so to speak), must carry his or her pocketbook
in his or her mouth, the hands being fully occupied
holding the gown together to avoid mooning the
assembly.

Here something must be said about the hospital
gown, for the benefit of the reader who has led a
sheltered life, sartorially, and doesn't understand that
this single garment can reduce a previously normal
person to a gibbering idiot who must be transferred
to the psychiatric ward. At first glance, nothing about
the hospital gown suggests that it has been exquisi-
tely designed to persuade the already nervous patient
that he has lost it mentally as well as physically. The
original, dating back to the Toga Period of imperial
Rome, was styled by the personal couturier to Julius
Caesar. After Caesar was stabbed to death by the
conspirators on the steps of the Senate, and his
slashed toga was shown to the mob, Mark Anthony –
and here I paraphrase Shakespeare – cried, "Look at
this awful bloody gown!" And that comment has
lived to this day.

Here are some of the features that have made the
hospital gown such a durable source of hysteria. First,
it must be worn back to front. The ties are at the back. It
is impossible to knot these ribbons unless you are the
sort of person who does reverse writing that can be
read with a mirror. Even if you have this special talent,
you will have difficulty tying the ribbons, since one (or
more) of them has been ripped off by a previous wearer
in a manic frenzy. When the hospital gown goes to the
laundry, it is checked, and if it still has any ties it is
thrown away as too easy.

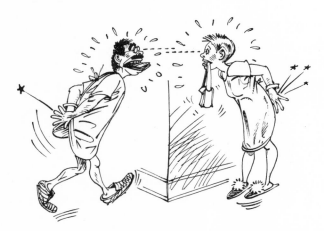

The first time I tried to knot the gown ties I went for
an elegant bow, initiating a period of colourful mono-
logue that explains the blistered paint on the walls of
the changing cubicle. I progressed rapidly into fashion-
ing a do-it-yourself straitjacket, complemented by a
half-nelson that made it hard for me to put my wallet
between my teeth. It was the sort of homespun
restrainer, cheaply made of available materials, that
might be of interest to the secret police of one of the
more impoverished Third World countries.

"Mr. Nicol?"

I was being winkled out of my cubicle. Ready or not,
here I come, and God help me if my aft-sail catches the
wind of the air-conditioning.

"How are you?" smiled the nurse, as though I might
be something other than mortified. Nurses are nice. I
have tremendous respect for nurses. My first wife was a
nurse. Also a nurse is my present, and almost certainly
last, wife. I am instinctively drawn to nurses because
they are lovely, caring women. (Male nurses I'm less
drawn to, no matter how lovely and caring they are; a

shameful admission, but there it is.) To this hospital nurse I said through my wallet:

"Do you come here often?"

She smiled again and ushered me into the cavernous room in the middle of which loomed, cryptic as Stonehenge, the great CAT. The male technician, Asian and impassive, took over my body, bidding me to recline on the narrow table, making sure that my head was comfy on the pillow. I got an insight into how Fay Wray felt when she was being prepared as the human sacrifice to King Kong. Toothsomely vulnerable while scared shitless.

The table slid me head first into the CAT, much as a torpedo is inserted into the firing-tube. My nose – a facial prominence suddenly placed at risk – cleared the barrel by less than an inch. The CAT hasn't got my tongue, but it came damn close to snagging the schnoz. How portly people fare when being ingurgitated by the machine, I hesitate to guess. Seems like a messy way to lose weight.

With my head projecting from one side of the CAT and my lower torso from the other, I remained very still while the technician instructed me:

"Watch the green light. When the light turns red, do not breathe. When the light turns green again, you may breathe. Do not move."

I heard his footsteps departing. We were alone, the green-eyed monster and I, as I knew we would be. I did not move. My flesh wanted to creep, but I wouldn't let it. Besides, there was nowhere for it to creep to. I kept my breathing shallow. Very shallow. My lungs must have thought I'd died. I thought about death. About my income tax. Anything to avoid giggling when the light turned red. . . .

Beep! The light turned red. I held my breath. Almost

immediately it turned green. Had I offended the CAT somehow? Bad breathless? The CAT grumbled to a new position in its surround of me. Beep. Red light. Hold breath. Green light. Yes, I was getting the hang of using the equipment. Years of training as a motorist helps.

Then the green light stayed on longer than at most intersections. The CAT remained immobile. Was this a trick? Was it trying to lull me into blinking – something I hadn't done since I dropped my shorts?

I heard voices, off. My eyes being frozen on the green light, I couldn't see where the voices were coming from, but they appeared human. Someone was, in fact, laughing. What had they seen on the screen to tickle their funny-bone? *My* funny-bone? Which the CAT had revealed to be not in my elbow but a tail wag?

No, it was the staff coffee break. I could distinguish a few words – "powder" . . . "fractured". . . Either the staff was reviewing a skiing weekend or the scan had shown that my back was broken and reduced to talc. Eventually the CAT's eye turned red. I was ready for it. A less alert patient might have allowed himself to be lulled into inattention, even a snooze. Not me. I can maintain an anxiety level longer than people half my age. The CAT rumbled and beeped, rumbled and beeped, again and again. I focussed my mind: it was a good thing I had not parked my car in a one-hour zone. This filming could take longer than *Gone With The Wind*. . . .

Maybe they left the best scenes on the cutting-room floor. Whatever, I was a bit disappointed when Dr. Goodbody let me look at a couple of the CAT scan pix. For one thing, they had shot me in black-and-white. Everybody knows that that dates you. Makes you look older. If TV can retouch Alfred Hitchcock in colour, why not make my spine look contemporary?

Worse, I couldn't grasp the plot. Dr. Goodbody tried to clarify:

"You can see the narrowing of the channel between the fourth and fifth vertebrae."

"Yeah, wow," I lied, not knowing the fourth and fifth vertebrae from Laurel and Hardy.

That was all he showed me. I had hoped – having spent so much quality time inside the CAT – that we might go through a whole album of pictures together. I didn't expect to see any smiling groups of discs, but it would have been nice to browse.

Still, I had seen something of my back without having to stand in front of a three-way mirror, a procedure that usually entails buying a new suit. As I hadn't bought a suit for forty years, it was a novelty to get a rear view of myself, though skeletal.

But Dr. Goodbody was not satisfied. He wanted me to have a myelogram *in addition* to the CAT scan and the ordinary X-rays. Surely, I thought, this risks overexposure, the thing that killed the Playboy clubs. Flattered though I was that my surgeon found my crumbling core to be a fund of fascinating frights needing to be documented, I almost wished that he were prepared to wing it a little. My impulse was to say:

"Let's go with what we've got, and take the chance that you'll hit hardpan."

I didn't, of course. He was just doing his job, being thorough enough to make me regret that I had not been referred to a neurosurgeon who approached my back operation the way he would a present found under the Christmas tree, just shaking me a couple of times before opening me up.

3

Myelogram – The Dye Is Cast

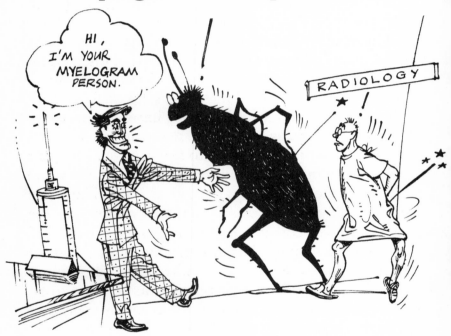

The back books advise against having a myelogram unless you are serious about surgery. If you are simply looking for a way to fill a couple of hours because the TV is into reruns, you would be better entertained, as a masochist, by going shopping for shoes a size too small for you.

Fortunately, the temptation to experience a new sensation is modified by the need to have authorization from your doctor. You can't just walk in off the street and tell hospital radiology: "I've got this awful crick in my neck. I'll take a myelogram – collar-size fifteen."

The myelogram is when you have to make up your mind whether you are going to fish or cut bait. I spent several months playing with the lure, reluctant to make that cast into murky waters. The decision had to be entirely mine. My wife, my children, my friends, the cat – none of them pressured me to get on with it. God, how I hated that! If I opted for the myelogram, and the intrusive needle went in a millimetre too far, I would have no one to blame but myself from my very own wheelchair. Detestable! Not only to spend the rest of my life as a human pretzel but to know that I had acted of my own free will – *that* stupid old thing.

Then I caught a break. The nurses in my province went on strike. Including those at the hospital where my myelogram would happen. To reach Radiology, I would have to cross the picket line. I have been a strong union man (Alliance of Canadian Television and Radio Artists) for years. I may not attend meetings, and sometimes I work for less than union scale, but I deeply respect the rights of my brothers – in this case sisters – of labour's federation. No way would I attempt to force a path through the placard-bearing ranks of those underpaid, overworked angels of mercy. The sciatic pain? Yes, I would find the strength to endure it, knowing that somewhere the spirit of Jimmy Hoffa was blessing me.

I was therefore appalled when the nurses' strike started to waver. The confounded provincial government leaned on the union to settle, despite the nurses' warning that, under the resultant stressed working conditions, patients were bound to suffer. Those that died, they implied, would be the lucky ones. And I knew exactly who would be the first patient to have his life placed in jeopardy because an exhausted nurse tossed her cigarette match into my oxygen tent. I was strongly tempted to attend the union meeting, standing outside the door and handing out pamphlets urging the nurses to reject the new agreement.

The picket line was down. My jig was up. Once more I found myself putting my clothes in a strange locker, to don the sacrificial robe. Sometimes the robe is blue, sometimes pink. Gender is no longer relevant. The patient has become an asexual being. If he or she doesn't make it, the transition to an eternal abode require no change of wardrobe. One size fits all souls.

A nurse escorted me into the concrete bunker in Radiology where the myelogram is performed. The room is in limbo, an almost Stygian darkness. People glide about me in the gloom – nurses, technicians, radiologists. Cryptic murmurs. I sense that I have become part of the cast for a Kafka play in which the protagonist is transformed into a cockroach.

A dark, handsome male teenager, incongruously

wearing a smart business suit, vested and necktied, comes to me and introduces himself. "I'm your myelographer," says he. Well, clearly he isn't a teenager after all. To a gaffer of my age, nearly all doctors and nurses look far too young to be entrusted with your body. So, I listen intently as this child explains what he proposes to do to me. Considerate of him, I think, till he finishes by presenting the consent form for me to sign. Oh, those halcyon days when the age of consent had to do with having sex! Now I consent to waiving grounds for a malpractice suit unless the doctor actually resorts to a chain-saw.

Having obtained my consent, the myelographer strolls away chatting to a comely blonde. Why, I muse, is he not wearing a white smock, like the doctors on the TV soaps? I know that it is now common for the family physician to eschew the uniform in his or her office, often being clad as though the patient's visit is the only thing between the doctor and the golf course. But *in the hospital*, damn it, the emotionally insecure patient deserves the visual assurance that the doctor *is* in fact an MD, complete with the stethoscope draped around the neck. I don't insist on them all wearing little mirrors on their foreheads, but to cruise around the wards looking like an ad in *Gentlemen's Quarterly* shatters the patient's conception of the trusty old Doc.

The doctor is, after all, a god-like figure. Just as the priest, when on duty, must be invested in his ritual surplice, and the judge must have his black gown and his wig to distance himself from the possibility of human error, so the doctor needs to accoutre himself in keeping with the awe in which he is held. I can't imagine the Supreme Being wearing a hand-tailored pinstripe suit, and I visualize the doctor also wearing the white smock, though not necessarily buttoned. The doctor can flap if he wishes. But smockless, and assisted by nurses who have abandoned the neat starched caps worn with short skirts and St. Trinian's stockings in favour of *pink slacks*, for God's sake, they convey the impression that they are merely human, like me. That's scary.

"Lie on the table, please." The myelogram nurse did not appear to be wearing a sweatsuit, though it was hard to tell in the murky chamber.

"On my stomach or my back?" The question had to be asked. I didn't wish to sound impertinent, but once I am on the buffet I hate to have to flip-flop, because my hospital gown always gapes and there goes my chance of dying with dignity. And as any bad-backer knows, turning over while lying down is not the easy move it once was. I have been tempted to ask, "Do you want me prone or supine?" But most medics don't know the difference ("Just lay there, ducky"). As for "prostrate," it sounds too much like "prostate" to be used anywhere near an operating-table.

"On your stomach, please," said the nurse.

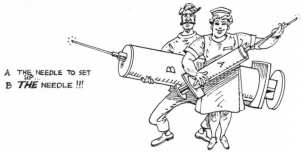

A THE NEEDLE TO SET
       UP...
B *THE* NEEDLE !!!

This was a switch. All the preceding X-rays of my back had placed me sunny side up, easy on the bacon. I was soon to learn why, like Milton's Satan cast down into Hell, I landed on my face. I heard the voice of the dapper male myelographer hovering above me, out of eyeshot. A quiet, reassuring tone:

"I'm going to give you an injection to desensitize the area of your back before I inject the dye."

Goody. A needle to set up *the* needle. With all this needlework I should end up with a back remarkable for its built-in quilt.

After a pause during which my dorsal nerves were rendered insensible, the gentle voice said, "Now I am going to inject the dye into the dural sac, the sheath around the spinal cord and nerve roots. . . ."

That sounded like fun too. Think of the dural sac as a sort of soda-pop straw, except that instead of a Slurpee you are sucking up dye.

" . . . The dye is a colourless liquid that is radio-opaque. That is, it blocks out X-rays. . . ." Lucky dye. "You may feel a slight chilling sensation. . . ."

I was glad not to be watching the process. They had not put a monitor where I could see it, but by the abrupt stillness of everyone in the room I knew that we had come to the part of the operation that I never watch on educational TV.

How does one describe the unique sensation of a needle piercing one's dural sac? The easy answer – "I guess you had to be there" – will not satisfy the reader who is trying to weigh the negatives of back surgery. Nor is it sufficient to mention that patients have been known to faint. Especially young men. Football players, steeplejacks, craven types like that, often swoon right there on the table, I was told, while elderly ladies keep right on chirping as though it's just another visit by the grandchildren.

Not painful, but weirdly sickening – that's how I'd describe the way the dye is cast. Like Caesar crossing the Rubicon, the patient has reservations about choosing this course unless turning back is *really* embarrassing. Anyway, the dye injection is not protracted. It's not like the ordinary service station where the attendant leaves the nozzle in your tank while he cleans the windshield. I doubt that I took more than four or five gallons before the hose was back on the hook.

"Now we're going to tilt you," advised a female voice. This explained why my feet rested against a flat board at the bottom of the table: to take my weight as I was raised, like a rocket-launcher. I braced myself for someone to bark "Fire One!"

Now poised almost perpendicular to the floor, I could glimpse the person who had last addressed me: the knock-down gorgeous blonde I had seen chatting with the male myelographer. Another doctor! Again my quaint, sexist conception of what a doctor looks like (Spencer Tracy) was shattered. I said to her:

"You made me rise to the occasion." In tense situations I have this remarkable ability to talk like a nerd. I was vaguely aware that the X-ray machine had been moved in behind my back, and other people were busy trying to focus its lethal rays on my verso, where anything out of place would show up against the background of the dye. The lady doctor sought to keep me from fretting. "We're going to have to tilt you some more."

"Roger," I said. "Had they started the countdown?"

She didn't appear to hear the question. It seemed that the ground crew working to my rear had run into a problem that was delaying my lift-off from the gantry. The lady doctor said, "Please keep your arms above your head." I raised my arms to the basic drugstore-holdup position. I surrender. The murmurs of frustration continued behind me. Although I had only one ear operational, I gathered that the dye was stubbornly defying the force of gravity supposed to make it flow down into the wonky segments of my spine. I heard the word "tight" muttered several times. What if they couldn't get the dye to seep through the debris? Would they tell me, "Sorry, but you'll have to call Roto-Rooter"? Or might I expect a second injection, this time nitroglycerine?

During one of the awkward silences that can blight a social affair, I attempted small talk with the blonde doctor. "Your hair is wet," I said, admiringly. "You are lovely when your hair is wet."

"I went for a swim before I came to work." She remained distracted by the problem that was making my arms ache above my head. "Could you turn slightly on your side?"

"Certainly," I said, rotating gingerly on the pad. At the same time I felt her hand on my bottom, propelling me, while her other hand braked me by pressing against my intromittent organ.

"Sorry!" Her apology was hasty but sincere, I regretted to note. She had already moved her hand to safer ground. Gone, my last chance to slip the surly bonds of Earth. The rest of my hour on the tilt-board was relatively uneventful, other than strengthening my impression that the myelogram team had met its match in my back, and wished that I had taken my business elsewhere.

Returned to the near-horizontal, I was summarily rolled onto a stretcher for despatch to Medical Day Care. "Drink plenty of fluids," a nurse advised, "to help flush the dye out of your system. And keep your head elevated for twenty-four hours."

I knew the purpose of these measures: to mitigate the effects of the myelogram, namely horrendous headaches if the dye is allowed to drift northward and pollute an already defiled mind. These headaches, though rare, are not exhilarating. One editor of my acquaintance opted for back surgery some days later on being assured that it would cure his myelogram headache. So, parked in the hall outside Radiology, I rested on my elbows and kept a sharp eye out for fluids. I gathered that eventually someone would come to push my gurney to Medical Day Care, where I would be awash in liquids.

Meantime, I was able to observe the flow of traffic through the busy intersection of hospital wings. Other patients, nurses, doctors, visitors, security people – a veritable medley of humanity – edged past me with that nervous glance people use when they are afraid they may see a corpse. I had ample time to learn that a person lying on a stretcher in a public thoroughfare is not only sexless and ageless, but well on the way to being lifeless. I took pains to ensure that the sheet shrouding my body was not drawn over my face. Even so, a couple of nurses in a nearby office nattered about intimate details of their love life, as though I was in a condition to hear nought but the summons of Valhalla's flugelhorn.

It was borne in upon me that the paths of glory lead but to the grave, and you can also stall on the exit ramp. The longer I lay there on the stretcher, the better I understood that the hospital-patient experience is an introduction to humility. This may be salutary for some (and I'm sure you can think of some worthy candidates), but not for the likes of fine people like you and me. Personally, if I want to eat humble pie, I'll ask to see the just-desserts menu.

At last an Asian chap popped out of a Radiology room to say to me: "Mr. Nichols?" It was close enough. I nodded. He said: "We have decided to give you a CAT scan. The machine is not being used." And he pushed me into a room where I goggled at a machine that looked like the mother of the one that had ingested me at the University Hospital.

"Excuse me," I babbled, "but I have already been scanned alive, by – "

"Don't move, please." He was not interested in how many times this marvellous X-ray colossus had diced my spine like the baked-ham slicer at the delicatessen. He went away, and I was alone once again with the big CAT. For twenty minutes. I had to conclude that whatever was wrong with my discs was taxing the capacity of every method of radiology known to modern science. Maybe, when I was a kid, I licked my pencil too often, building up a lead shield around my spine that the machines, superbly sophisticated though they were, found impenetrable. Maybe I was making medical history. Would get written up in *Time* – "CANADIAN'S BACK DEFIES DIAGNOSTIC SCIENCE". . . . The *New England Journal of Medicine* would devote an issue to me. Fame at last!

I was back in the corridor again. Lying on the same stretcher. Waiting to be moved to Medical Day Care. From my reading I knew that there were still several other diagnostic X-rays that I could be subjected to, if the machine was not being used. The *discogram*, for example, said to be quite painful for the patient but something of a romp for the radiologist. And the *epidural venogram*, in which the radiopaque fluid is injected into veins in the groin and flows *upward* into the spine, with unscheduled stops at points of interest. And the *epiduragram*, where the dye is injected not inside but *outside* the dural sac, to outline any bulging discs, lost car keys, or other bric-à-brac that has got lodged in the lumbar region.

If I were pregnant, of course, I could also qualify for ultrasound, a non-invasive technique, but I'm afraid there's no womb on my dance card.

Also on the radioactive *carte du jour*: bone scanning, nerve-root injection, facet injection . . . Golly, everything looks so inviting, I just can't make up their mind.

A large woman in white hove out of the stream of people ignoring me on the stretcher. "Mr. Nicole?" She gave it the French accent, to rhyme with "geek hole." I didn't quibble.

"Thank God you've found me. Are we still at war with Japan?"

Impassive, she swung around behind my head, and the stretcher began to move, briskly, through the busy intersection. We appeared to have the right of way, but where was the green light when I needed it?

"You're taking me to Medical Day Care," I said, trying not to sound nosy. From the grunt behind my left ear I inferred that Medical Day Care was indeed our destination and that my propeller did not see getting there as half the fun.

Before I was finally dismissed by the hospital, months later, I was to take a half-dozen of these whirlwind tours of the complex. It was only when I watched the Winter Olympics on TV and saw the luge event from a camera strapped on the stomach of a competitor that I realized that I had been here before. In terms of hapless hurtling around corners and from one level to another on the flat of the back, the luge is only a colder open-air version of stretcher travel around the average hospital. Called "Transport," the sturdy women who provide the propulsion have the steely-eyed mien – the Paul Newman look – of Formula One drivers every-where. They don't say much. They let the wheels do the talking. And I got the message ("Get him there before he dies on your shift") very quickly.

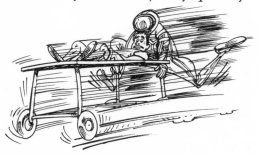

Staring through the gun-sight V of my own feet as we barrelled along, I watched walls whiz by, steel doors smash open before our battering-ram, and other stretchers and laundry carts scream on two wheels out of our way. Above, the writhing patterns of steam pipes on tunnel ceilings were interrupted by pit stops in elevators hurriedly emptied by visitors anxious not to be trapped in a confined space with a body that might be still infectious.

The reception for me in the Medical Day Care ward – a vast room whose walls were lined with beds, redolent of the old "Carry On, Doctor" type of farce that the Brits used to film – was informal. But I was on my guard. I didn't want to be drawn into a "Carry On" routine like:

SURGEON (on rounds): And what's your trouble?

MALE PATIENT: Well, this grenade went off between me legs, and –

SURGEON: Ah, rectum?

MALE PATIENT: Well, it didn't do 'em any good.

I was watchful for the fun-loving nurse who, on the pretence of administering an enema, left me lying prone with a daffodil inserted in my orifice.

By now the reader will know me well enough to understand that I have an irrational fear of being para-noid. I attribute my bad back in part to having leaned over backwards too often. One of my objects in doing so is to avoid having people such as doctors and nurses point at me and whisper, "That man is schizy. Send him up to Psych Ward for a couple of jolts of reality." Fore-most among my nightmares has been that of finding myself a patient in a large ward with multiple strangers with whom I have nothing in common but mortality. All my plans for survival have been built around having a private room. With a private bathroom. And a private nurse. To whom I can explain, privately, exactly why privacy is essential to a person who always sleeps with a pillow over his head and farts *con brio*.

I was therefore surprised at how quickly I adjusted to the Medical Day Care room. The fact that I was in no pain whatever, while others around me were bleeding visibly from wounds, moaning, or simply lying unconscious, doubtless made me feel more compan-ionable. One or two had the curtain drawn around their beds, which is carrying privacy too far. Some had to go pot in the cot. Not me. Fully ambulant (a medical term meaning "able to limp about"), and drinking fluid in such quantity as to carry the myelogram dye out of my system in a tidal wave of wee-wee, I made it to the communal washroom every few minutes. I was glad that I had worn knee-length socks. A male patient publicly padding about in ankle socks looks ridiculous, in my opinion. His knees may be tanned, but his sucking in his belly for the nurses is effectively cancelled out by his exposing scrawny, pallid shanks that only a mother could love.

After your myelogram, you can expect to be kept in Medical Day Care for four to six hours; longer, if you make the mistake of complaining that your head is asking for a divorce from your neck, or if you wander around the ward wild-eyed, pointing to your wound and quoting Mercutio: " 'Tis not so deep as a well, nor so wide as a church door, but 'tis enough, 'twill serve. . . .' "

I was ready, nay panting, for parole after only three hours. Every hour a nurse came to take the vital signs that I was to recognize as my passport to freedom. I soon learned to read the chart that kept me prisoner, and to appreciate the hefty, unattractive nurse, since she was less apt to send my temperature and blood pressure soaring than the registered knockout, leaning over me with her exuberant bosom.

There are so many pretty nurses in our hospitals that the male patient should be prepared to either close his eyes and stop his ears every time one of these beauties ministers to him, or land up in Intensive Care.

In Medical Day Care, one of my nurses cheekily tweaked my big toe, en passant. I didn't know how to respond. Coupled with the blonde radiologist's unsolicited fondling of another of my appendages, this added up to more casual sex than I had enjoyed since I played Musical Chairs in kindergarten. My considered opinion is that female nurses *relish* taking advantage of men who are temporarily unable to repel liberties like toe-tweaking, lap-tapping, shoulder-squeezing, and cheek-patting. No actual crude sexual assault. But a lot of this good-natured teasing can result in a man's lying under a tent, regardless of whether he had it in mind to go camping.

After waiting eight hours in Medical Day Care, I wanted to wave a sign reading REMEMBER ME? At last the dapper teenage radiologist sauntered into the ward, glanced at my chart, and said, "How do you feel?"

"Great!" I replied. "Never better. I've been voiding like the Bay of Fundy. Have kept my head raised. Completely drained . . ."

"Wiggle your feet," he said.

I wiggled them frantically. The doctor nodded, handed the chart to a nurse, and left. The nurse yanked my curtain closed so that I could scramble into my clothes. Free! Free! Everyone should spend some time in hospital so that he or she can relate more closely to Nelson Mandela. I emerged from behind my curtain with the panache of a Ziegfeld Follies star taking her bows. I blew kisses to the nurses, none of whom noticed. "Toodle-oo" I carolled. "Also adieu!" I felt good enough to indulge biculturalism.

"Hold it," said the head nurse, before I could nip past her station. "Somebody's picking you up?"

"No, ma'am," I said blithely. "I drove myself to the hospital. I'm driving myself home. Asta la vista! . . ."

"Not so fast, Mr. Nicol. We don't normally allow patients to drive right after a myelogram. I'll have to get the okay from the doctor." She picked up the phone. I knew I was looking at another eight hours.

"No, no, please!" I pleaded. "I promise to drive defensively. I'll stay on the sidewalk . . ."

To no avail. Never try to argue with a head nurse. One might as well try to budge Boulder Dam. I sat and waited till the doctor responded to his pager and – after some discussion from which I was excluded – granted the pardon. I could be my own chauffeur. As I walked to the parking-lot, I realized that all of this had destroyed my self-confidence in my ability to operate a vehicle. Was I, in fact, now developing a myelogram headache, which would climax as I was attempting to outwit a yellow light? Did I trip over that curb because the doctors had erred in assuming that my brain was at the top end of my spine?

I am not suggestible. I just don't trust myself to feel confident.

Rush-hour traffic. I edged the Honda into it gingerly. Perhaps I should have put a sign in the back window: STUNNED DRIVER. Too late now. I have to have faith in the sensitivity of other motorists to recognize that a fellow mortal is recovering from an invasive diagnostic procedure, which is why he is driving at 20 km/h. With his distress signals blinking.

Few did. I absorbed a revelatory lesson in how little empathy prevails among the motoring public. The same person who, to help the elderly person walk across the street, will give him a hand, can spare only one finger when the oldster sits behind the wheel. Nor does it mitigate the hostility, I found, to point appealingly at your back and mouth the word "myelogram." The guy leaning on the horn takes it as an exotic form of obscene gesture and goes into a frenzy. Try it some time when your car doors are securely locked.

Civilization ends at the turn of key in ignition.

Having made it safely to within a block of my house,

I put on a burst of speed (30 km/h) to retrieve something of my chutzpah, and made a Grand Prix entrance into the garage, taking out a few garden tools.

"How did it go?" asked my wife.

I flashed her a Douglas Fairbanks Jr. smile. "Piece of cake."

"The myelogram didn't bother you?"

"Does the sugaring-off bother the maple tree? So they stick a funnel in your trunk and collect the sap. Big deal. Fancy waffles for dinner?"

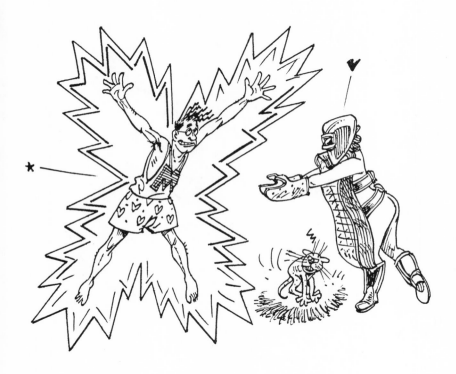

4

The Price of Admission

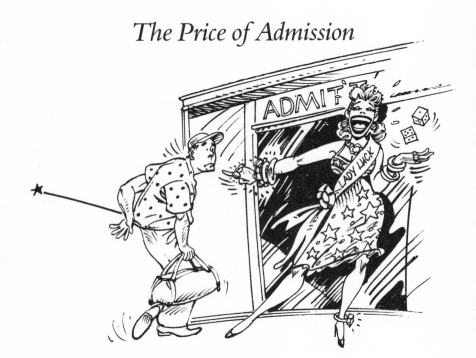

Dr. Goodbody phoned to tell me the results of my screen test. He liked what he saw. "It's a great myelogram," he said.

"You mean it's a horror film."

"That's right. Between two and three it's tight. Three and four, tighter. Between four and five it's *really* tight."

It was not the first time I have been called tight. But previously it was my pocket that was affected. It didn't take a neurosurgeon to open it up, and my children's stories about the need for a local anesthetic are grossly exaggerated.

Dr. Goodbody was waiting for me to respond to his confirming that my discs were tighter than Glasgow on a Saturday night. It was the moment of truth. Again. I could do with a few more moments of pure speculation. I have to give the surgeon the go-ahead, or live the rest of my life with a progressively pinched nerve that pretty well eliminates any hope of my dancing the limbo. Either way, the opportunity for major grief is rife. Maybe I should delay the decision till I have consulted a reliable soothsayer . . . had a few voodoo priests examine chicken entrails . . . hell, at least had my teacup read . . .

"Okay, doctor, let's go for it." I was astounded to hear myself say it. Surely this was some kind of ventriloquism, my alter ego butting in where I and angels fear to tread.

"Right. I'll set it up." The line went dead.

I replaced the receiver thoughtfully. You mad,

impetuous fool, I told myself, what have you *done*? You own a nice, unscarred back, silky skin admired in the past by ladies whose fingers plied the region. You want to try for washboard?

The phone had scarcely cooled from my hand before I began hearing from people – family members, friends, complete strangers who stopped me on the street – with grisly tales to tell about persons they knew who had had back surgery.

"Oh, wow," cautioned my daughter, gazing at me as though I was already panhandling on a skateboard. "Some bikers I know had back surgery . . ." Her voice trailed off. But I got the message. Those big, strong guys, after their surgery, traded in their Harley for a walker. Their beards turned white, and their shades are now those of the legally blind. The dragon tattooed on their biceps has shrunk to an earthworm with an attitude problem.

Every time I opened a newspaper or magazine I was confronted by an article headed something like BACK SURGERY WITHOUT STITCHES. I read about chymopopain – a *painless* pain. The doctor injects a derivative of the pawpaw into the herniated disc, where it acts like a meat tenderizer on a $2 steak and gobbles up the stray bits that are hurting you, like an internal Pacman. I've always fancied the pawpaw since I first discovered the fruit while honeymooning in Fiji. However, my enthusiasm for the pawpaw is not shared by our conservative Canadian physicians. To get a referral to a practitioner of chemonucleolysis seemed to me to be almost as hard as pronouncing it. I decided not to second-guess my own doctor. Politically I'm an anarchist, but when it comes to the government of my body, I am right-wing to the point of being downright fascist.

Still, I felt queasy when I opened my copy of *Time* magazine and saw in the Medicine section a glowing piece on a revolutionary procedure called percutaneous automated diskectomy. On syllable count alone, this operation outranked my decompressive laminectomy. Better yet, I would be an outpatient – the very best kind of patient you can be without having your operation faxed to you. The PAD requires no general anesthetic, merely a thin steel tube sneaked into the doleful disc, to admit a wee cutting/suction device the diameter of a pencil lead that slices and aspirates the offending material with less disturbance to the patient than having Sears in to clean the carpets.

"Patients walk out of the hospital with only a Band-Aid over the incision," marvelled *Time*. No painkiller needed except an Aspirin or two and Mummy to kiss it better. Back to work in a week. A scar invisible to even the most powerful American spy satellites.

Why wasn't *I* being siphoned? The article said that the procedure has a high success rate (four out of five cases), being unsuitable only for discs that have blown their contents so completely, created so much rubble, that not even a built-in vacuum system can clean them up.

Such, obviously, was my case. Not for me the PAD T-shirt inscribed SURGERY SUCKS. For me it will be something more akin to drilling for oil in the Beaufort Sea. . . .

My mind sought solace in what my family doctor had said that was most memorable: "You can always cancel the surgery." What an inspiration those words were! During the weeks of waiting for The Call, I included that mantra in my bedtime prayer: " . . . and if I should die before I wake, please cancel the surgery."

In the morning I said to my wife: "By golly, the sciatica in my legs seems less today. I think I'll cancel the surgery."

"I saw you limping to the bathroom."

"I was doing my Hopalong Cassidy impression."

"And now you are standing with one foot on the cat."

"She likes it." Mind over matter. As dominatrices go, a limp whip. Just when I had mustered enough self-delusion to cancel the operation, I got a little reminder that rubbing the belly of the small Buddha beside my bed had not solved the problem. For instance, in the supermarket queue, I was the only person with one leg hung over the handle of the cart. Having one foot dangling among the frozen cranberry juice can give you a nasty case of frostbite.

Worse, one of my daughters got married, and I had to stand at the altar to give the bride away, because they wouldn't let me work from a squat. I kept giving the minister the TV hurry-up sign, which he normally gets only when the bride is very pregnant. Made him nervous. No question, I detracted from the solemnization by suddenly sitting on the groom's mother's lap.

Then, suddenly, and as though I never expected it, early one Monday morning in January my phone rings. The caller has such a sweet voice, so disarming . . .

"Good morning, Mr. Nicol. It's Dr. Goodbody's secretary. . . ." It is impossible to recognize it as the summons of Destiny. " . . . We have a bed for you."

I wanted to tell her, nicely, that I already had a bed, thanks. My own little truckle bed. Under which I should have hidden the instant the phone rang. Too late now. She is continuing: "Can you come into the hospital this afternoon?"

This *afternoon*? *This* afternoon? The post meridiem of this very day? A matter of hours, for the arrival by a person for whom foot-dragging is not only a symptom of his bad back but a factor in requiring an ETA measured in weeks, possibly months? The doctor's secretary went on:

"The doctor has scheduled your surgery for tomorrow morning. The hospital likes you to be there the day before, for preparation."

What preparation? How long does it take to paint a bull's-eye on a guy's back? I quavered: "How long have I got?"

"Admitting likes you to be there before three. I suggest between one and two."

"Four hours from now." The words crawl from a mouth turned Sahara. Four hours in which to put my affairs in order. A piddling 240 minutes, to wash my hair, make my peace with God, pack . . .

"Mr. Nicol?"

"I'm still here." She expected an answer. The situation was an echo of the exquisite Jack Benny moment when a gunman says to him, "Your money or your life." Like Benny, I wanted more time to weigh the options.

It would have been dead easy to lie, to tell the secretary, "Oops, I forgot – my wife and I are flying to Hawaii this week. Damn, I'll have to postpone the operation. I can't disappoint Mrs. Nicol. She has her heart set on a beach boy . . ."

No, the secretary will know I'm fibbing. Even over the phone she'll sense the lengthening of my beak. . . .

"Okay. I'll be there."

I hung up. My heart was pounding. I couldn't blame it. *I'd* be furious too, if some old fool was dragging me into surgery that would be a hell of a lot more stressful than a normal test, such as watching the Miss Universe pageant.

As soon as I could control my vocal cords, down from a squeak, I told my wife I had a bed. She was elated. "Isn't that wonderful?" she cried. "At last you can get it over and done with."

Over and Donewith. Sounded like the name of a funeral home. I feigned delight. "Marvy," I said.

"I'll drive you to the hospital."

Thanks, I'll walk. Preferably by way of Monaco.

Something in my manner told her that my joy was not altogether unmitigated. Her eyes filled and she embraced me. "My brave darling," she said.

What a hideous thing to say! Here I am aching to be supported as the devout coward I am, and my own wife strikes the white flag from my hand, substituting the standard of Joan of Arc. My wife has this habit of looking on the bright side. It drives me crazy.

"Everything," she said, "is going to be all right."

I wanted a second opinion. Mine. *My* opinion was that the Head Croupier in the celestial Vegas had pushed the dice into my sweaty palm, saying, "Roll 'em!" Here I was putting my life on the line, knowing that as a gambler I was not even distantly related to the man who broke the bank at Monte Carlo. I have long ago given up lottery and raffle tickets, and have been excommunicated from church bingo because I cast such a pall as a Jonah that nobody would sit near me. So what makes me think that I can beat the odds of major surgery?

Reliable statistics tell us that for hospital patients the chances are fifty/fifty that they will come out (if at all) in worse shape than when they went in. With my record in flirting with Lady Luck, those odds guaranteed that I would emerge with a tag on my toe, accompanied by a request that in lieu of flowers donations be sent to the Canadian League of the Jinxed.

"Thank you, my dear," I told my radiant wife. "I'll show you where I keep my will."

For some, putting their affairs in order consists mainly of telling their secretary that the dirty weekend is off, indefinitely. Not for me. I sat down heavily at the desk in my den and typed an advisory for my wife, listing all my investments and where they could be found, besides my piggy bank. I drew a map for her to locate the trust company named as co-executor of my will ("Ask for Colin – he's the one with the honest moustache"). And I jotted down a few touching but dignified suggestions for epitaphs for my tombstone, till I remembered I'd left instructions to be cremated and scattered on the rhubarb.

Packing was dead easy. I had already made the list: toothbrush and paste, electric shaver (without cord), dressing-gown, earplugs (hospitals can be a zoo at night), and a Woody Allen book, in case Norman Cousins was right, and laughing *can* divert the Grim Reaper. I also packed a work scribbler, to make notes for this book, on the premise that if an apple a day keeps the doctor away, a giggle or two pops you into the loo. For some reason I envisioned myself sitting up comfortably in my hospital bed, scoffing up grapes and knocking off one-liners that would earn robust royalties, after the book had been selected by the Hoot-of-the-Month Club.

In the post-op event, I couldn't even reach the drawer of the bedside table to fetch forth pencil and paper. Such notes as I was able to scrawl, on scraps of facial tissue and the palm of a hand, proved to be as difficult to decipher as a Mayan grocery list – and about as funny. If you really want to keep a day-to-day record of your hospital experience, you'd better have a tape-recorder implanted in your chest.

Another major hazard of the hospital room, one that my daughter warned me about after recovering from a Caesarean, is daytime television. Being in hospital for as long as a week, conscious enough to watch TV yet too weak to change channels as a parade of foot fetish-ists, child-molesters, and other assorted freaks strut their stuff on the talk shows – it's a terrifying prospect. Soap operas! Rife with death scenes in hospitals! A person could suffer irreparable brain damage.

However, the clock told me that I was too pressed for an inoculative shot of *The Young and the Restless*. I would just have to hope that my system was strong enough to absorb scenes of sexy young people doing things in bed that could protract my local bleeding.

My wife dropped me off, with my ditty-bag, at the hospital. I walked to the door. It was locked. Was God trying to tell me something? No, it was the wrong door. I found the main entrance and the lobby, a large space with no arrows pointing to anything that looked like Admitting. The Information desk was not manned, or womaned, or affording any living being that showed above the counter. Maybe this Informa-tion desk was like the one at international airports: a row of video display terminals with answers to every question except where do I go to meet Aunt Ida arriv-ing from Singapore?

Staying clear of Information, I intercepted a young

man whose blue shirt and intercom bespoke Security. "Excuse me, where do I make an admission?"

"To doing what?" he said, suspicious.

"Getting into the hospital. I want to take a bed." I waved my bag vaguely, as proof of intent to register.

Security pointed to the rear of the lobby, where I did indeed find a small sign ADMITTING. Beyond it, a smallish room. Crammed with people. Some – relatives and friends of the potentially deceased – stood in the crowded corridor. Others occupied a row of booths where admitting clerks extracted life histories from people like me who had hoped to die without revealing anything. Beyond the booths lay the bullpen of the waiting, seated elbow to elbow, with their pitiful personal effects, and even more pitiful personal defects.

Admitting is the great leveller. No doubt there are a few exalted persons – the CEO of General Motors, members of the Royal Family, people who own their own hospital – who are not required to go through the common process of admitting. But the rest of us, rich and poor, young and old, other-hued and white, must do our time in this congested oubliette that gives us a clearer idea of conditions in the Conciergerie during the Terror of the French Revolution.

I found a seat beside a young man who immediately got up from *his* seat and went to stand against the wall. My God, did I look *that* contagious? A bad back is not a transmittable disease. Yet he had taken one look at me and seen hepatitis A to Z. I have had this kind of thing happen to me in the movie theatre – the woman seated next to me getting up and moving to another row – but hell, in this waiting-room I wasn't even eating popcorn with my usual gusto.

Hurt, I nursed my bag on my lap and kept my eyes

on the nurse who had taken my name and promised to call me, though she didn't say during what paleozoological era.

After she left for her coffee break, I turned my attention to my fellow inmates, to try to guess what physical or mental affliction had brought each of them to this chamber of diagnosed horrors. The young looked impatient. They clearly resented the unkind fate that had marooned them with a conclave of crocks. Where there wasn't even the solace of a background rock band – the musical staff of life for anyone under thirty. Should I hum something? No. They don't look in the mood for "Oh, What a Beautiful Morning!"

The Asians looked, as usual, inscrutable. It was impossible to tell which was the patient and which the supporting relatives, on hand in numbers to translate, lest their beloved granny be whisked into Obstetrics instead of Extended Care.

The Hispanic couple was more animated. They appeared to be discussing, passionately, the question of which of them should be admitted. I'd have thought that they would have settled this matter before coming to the hospital, but then I know that as an Anglo-Saxon I lack spontaneity.

Finally, there were the aging loners, like me. Feigning insouciance. Que sera sera. I've lived a good life, folks, and if this is how it ends, hell, Hemingway stuck a shotgun in his mouth, but I'm willing to leave it to hospital food.

All of us look a little ashamed to be there. Your presence in Admitting is a confession that you have not taken proper care of the temple that is your body, may in fact have used it as a garbage dump. A person hospitalized by the wounds of war can feel honourable, unless he deliberately shot his toe off. I wish I had worn my WW II medals and blue beret. Too late now. The younger people have me tabbed as a psychopathic . . . the Asians as syphilitic . . . the Latins as dead.

"Mr. Nicol?" I lurch to an Admitting clerk's cubicle as her previous admission eases himself into a wheelchair. I'm shocked to see a person who has walked into Admitting under his own power (such as it is) already slouched in a wheelchair to be taken to his room. What kind of questions do they ask in this innocent-looking booth? Did the Admitting clerk take her training with the KGB? Is this what the hospital does to you? In case you are in any doubt about the seriousness of your condition, bingo, into the wheelchair? I could practically feel the draft of icy air mounting from the Morgue.

Having watched the dour departure of my predecessor, I sat down to have *my* history taken. History has never been my best subject. Especially my own history. I have a fairly firm grasp on the date of my birthday, but after that, my history tends to become anecdotal, not to say apocryphal. . . .

"How old are your children?" asks the Admitting clerk. A dreadful question to ask a man under stress. I know that I have three children. Tops. The number is fast in my mind. If I forget it, momentarily, all I have to do is think Holy Trinity, or Three Little Pigs. But my kids' ages? That involves subtracting three different sets of numbers, which change every year. I know it sounds sexist, but making these calculations is women's work. I have female friends and neighbours who can tell me at once, exactly, and without using a calculator, how old my children are because *their* children went to school with them and they know from memory how old their children are. From memory! I call it an unhealthy pre-occupation with chronology.

But I didn't say so to the Admitting clerk. I gave her three ballpark figures for my children's ages, and we moved on to other unwarranted personal questions.

"Do you have any diseases?"

They're asking *me*? Why am I here, in this enormous hospital, if not to establish the extent of my being diseased? That is why I pay medical insurance – to be told how many things are wrong with me.

"No," I replied. Later I realized that I lied. Among my diagnosed ills are a double hernia, non-allergenic vasomotor rhinitis, a tortuous bowel (too kinky to get a G rating), occasional prostatitis, and one suspicious mole. Why these anomalies slipped my mind, I don't know. I guess a person tries to put his best foot forward, regardless of whether the arch has fallen.

"Do you smoke?" This was the biggie. The $64,000 question, adjusted for inflation. I have never smoked in my life, but in the course of my hospitalization so many people asked me if I smoked – and here their eyes narrowed with scepticism – that I started wishing I had a cigarette. If only to chew. So, if you, the reader, are a smoker, it may not be worth your while to have elective surgery, unless of course to have a fag removed from your fingers. You will have to go outside the hospital to have a smoke, which you may rue if your wheelchair doesn't have snow tires and a blizzard blows you out of the parking-lot.

I gathered that if a hospital worker gets a whiff of the weed on your breath, your status automatically goes from stable to critical. You may be tossed into the oxygen tent before you can get your shoes off.

My dossier completed, the clerk sealed on my right

wrist the plastic name-band, my main protection against being wheeled into the O.R. for a hysterectomy, while Mrs. Blivitz gets my laminectomy. The wrist-band is the first tangible proof that I am registered property of the pest-house. Not my choice as a charm bracelet, the wristband is rather too much a constant reminder that at critical moments I shall be unable to say who I am, let alone where I am, why I am there, or which horse looks good in the fifth race.

I declined the wheelchair to transport me to my room. There may have been a touch of bravado in the way I waved off the wheels. Like refusing the blindfold before the firing-squad. But I tried not to make a meal of it, merely adding, "And never mind a porter – I can carry my bag myself." (I wasn't sure whether I would be expected to tip.) "Just point me in the direction of my room."

"You're in Room 502, East Five C."

"No problem." I gave her a swashbuckling smile. Fifteen minutes later, the smile had unbuckled its swash – I was lost. Traipsing from nursing-station to nursing-station. Quietly cursing the room-numbering system that was utterly alien to a man trained in that of cheap motels. Lost, and risking snow-blindness from staring at so many white uniforms, plus a mild hypo-thermia from frosty looks when I tried to find shelter in Gynecology.

Room 502 was a private room that was not really private. That is, it was too small to meet the standards of the true private, yet was a large enough closet to contain a bed, on a floor strapped for space. I had asked for a private room in hopes of getting some writing done without disturbing a room-mate with the teeth-grinding that sometimes accompanies my creativity.

The closet did have its own lavatory, however, a chamber that was to prove to be a blessed grotto second only to Lourdes. There are times, during your stay in hospital, when the toilet occupied by someone else looms as the major tragedy in your life. Divorce, loss of job, death of a loved one – traumatic, yes, but trivial compared to facing a locked john. For the hospital patient, as with the airline passenger, there can be times when the will to live teeters dangerously, and none more parlous than when he or she seeking the throne grasps the unyielding knob that says, "Thou shalt not enter the kingdom."

The other major disadvantage of the two- or four-bed room is that if, like me, you expect to have few visitors, it can be mortally depressing to be the only patient in the room who demonstrably has no one who cares a damn whether he recovers or hops the twig. When three other patients have visitors nattering away and plying them with bonbons, I find that the only way to escape total ignominy is to lie very still with the eyes closed, and the sheet drawn over your head, holding your breath till you hear a visitor whisper, "Oh, dear, I think Bed Four is . . . er . . . may be . . . passed away." That should quiet down the cheery chatter, and get you the curtain drawn, minimum.

Alternatively, if you really feel strongly about having visitors to boost your morale, it may be advisable, before entering the hospital, to join a club or a church group that has a hospital-visit committee. Then one or more members will visit you as a merciful act that earns them Brownie points with Providence. Becoming a Baptist may be the only way you'll see flowers in water, instead of a wreath. Or cookies to supplement the swill. Once you have been discharged from the hospital, you can reject the faith and return to your normal sab-bath of NFL football or major-league baseball.

Having stowed my gear in the locker, and hidden my wallet so that I would forget where I put it, I lay on the bed to await developments. The room did not have a chair. I learned later that this is normal. Chairs get pinched from vacant rooms, sometimes while the body is still warm. If *you* want a chair, for the visitor who isn't going to come, you should use this prelude period to nip out into the hall and scrounge a chair from a patient who appears to be in a coma.

Another tip: keep your street clothes on as long as possible. At some point during the prelude period a nurse will enter your room and toss onto your bed what looks like souvenirs of The Ragpickers' Ball. Ignore them. Also pay no attention to her instruction to put them on your body. These are hospital-patient gar-ments. Once you commit your mortal frame to that vestment, you are dressed in the same sense that a chicken is dressed. All you need is the stuffing. There-fore, postpone removing your street clothes as long as you can, even if it means tying extra knots in your shoelaces. The longer you can put off looking like a *fully institutional inmate*, in unisex gown and suicide-proofed slippers, the better your chances of negotiating with the nursing-station for such creature comforts as a pillow, blankets, or a call-button that works.

Naive fool that I was, I jumped into the hospital uniform right away and lay on the bed waiting for something to happen. The hospital bed is one of the hardest objects known to man. The mattress is made by people who apprenticed as stonemasons, and has roughly the same bounce as the Appalachian Shield. The slab is shrink-wrapped in heavy, slithery plastic to protect it from the patient's wayward juices. It can cause a feverish patient to hallucinate that he is adrift on an ice floe. I never felt closer to a seal pup.

True, I had a window bed. If things got really sticky, post-op, I wouldn't have to crawl over other patients in order to achieve defenestration. Meantime, the view of the hospital yard, of nurses and doctors and other staff going about their business, gave my ego a douche. How depressing, that life goes on, regardless of our peril, of our personal, possibly terminal, crisis! Why aren't all those people huddled beneath my window, gazing upward with grief-stricken faces? I don't expect an all-night vigil, with bulletins posted on the hospital gates, but, hell, not so much as a passing glance?. . .

A nurse came into my room. Young and pretty. Things were looking up. To hell with that cold world outside. Here was a care-giver. She fetched a chair, sat down, crossed her legs, and poised a clipboard on her lap.

"I've come to take your history," she said.

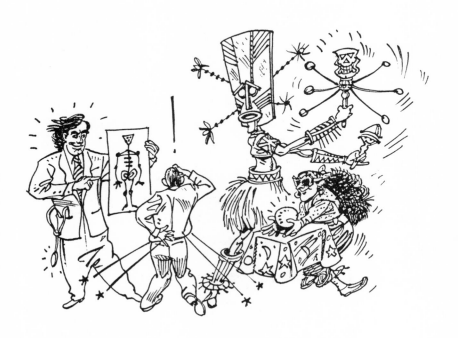

5

Night of the Green Berets

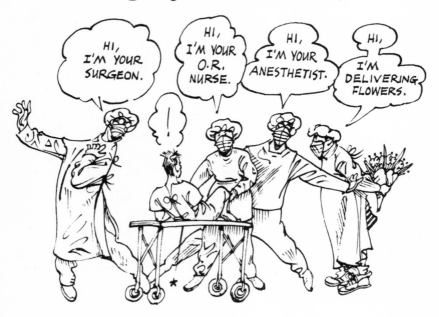

I should have asked for copies of all my histories taken that day. They would have fattened this account to two, possibly three, volumes. Of course, none of the histories were exactly the same. For instance, I soon grew weary of the question "How did you hurt your back?" With repetition, my reply – "I probably just wore it out playing badminton" – became a crashing bore. I didn't see an enquirer actually yawn, but it was obvious that the chronicle of my life was no threat to The Happy Hooker, or even Poor Mrs. Quack.

"I hurt my back as an airman during World War II, parachuting into occupied Belgium after a dog-fight. . . ." No. The eve of major surgery is no time to be inviting God's wrath by fibbing to impress a nurse because she has sky-blue eyes. Ordinarily I am not a believer in the Recording Angel and post-mortem judgment on high, but there are no atheists in the trenches or in Room 502. *After* the operation has proved successful, yes, if she still wants to know me better, I did hurt my back when my 'chute failed to open plummeting into the Ardennes forest. . . .

The pretty nurse left with my rheumatic résumé, and another nurse came to take my blood. Not all of it, but enough to make her competitive with the northern Saskatchewan mosquito. I never watch when my blood is taken. I keep up a lively if nervous chatter – "How are things in Transylvania? . . . I hope the garlic on my breath doesn't bother you. . . ." – but my eyes are fixed on an object in the middle distance, such as the end of my nose. I knew why I was being tapped – they wanted to identify my blood type in case something went haywire during the surgery and they had to give me a blood transfusion. Why didn't they just *ask* me? Having once been a blood donor, when I was young and able to afford a pint of transmission fluid, I could have told them that my blood was Type A. Or was it Type O? Somewhere between A and Z, definitely. Anyway, it was red.

Had I wanted to be *au courant*, I should have opened a savings account at the blood bank, to be drawn on if my regular account came up NSF. This is said to be the best way to avoid receiving blood of which the politest that may be said is that you don't know where it's been. But I'm not sure that my own blood is a keeper. It *looks* all right, on the rare occasions when a capillary condescends to bleed. But if I could be sure that I was getting plasma from a young, virile, heterosexual person with a good tennis backhand and an aversion to drugs, well, I'd be prepared to take my chances.

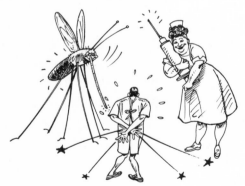

The sanguinary nurse departed with whatever she had managed to suck out of my arm, to be replaced by a tall gentleman who introduced himself as my anesthetist. I had never met an anesthetist before. Not in a long and reasonably full life. I had been introduced to a lot of people who put me to sleep, mostly at committee meetings. But none of them was a professional. They just had a knack, a gift of language. The kind of sedation they administered was too unregulated for any surgery except cutting short my attention span.

The anesthetist asked me a number of questions to see if I was breathing. And, if so, was it just a lucky try. "Do you smoke?" he asked. He obviously didn't trust any of the other histories I had fabricated. A fleck of Player's on my lip, and he'd be long gone.

"No, sir, I have never smoked." I said it with wonderment, as if discovering this marvellous fact about myself for the first time. "Both my parents smoked when I was a kid. My mother smoked cigarettes in a long, black holder, since it was the flapper era. I hated that black cigarette-holder. The smoke attracted men. I was jealous. I never got over seeing tobacco as a rival for my mother's affections. . . . "

The anesthetist's eyes were glazing over. Before he left, he reminded me that I was not to eat or drink anything after dinner, in preparation for the morrow's festivities. I knew that this fasting was a precaution against my tossing my bickies at the height of the operation, with possibly fatal consequences. Hospitals do not want the patient to throw up till you are fully alert and able to smell what the kitchen has sent you for breakfast.

For my dinner (which was to prove to be my last food for a week), the entrée was roast pork. Or it may have been roast chicken. Hospital kitchens have the technological know-how to cook every kind of meat so that it looks and tastes like any other kind of meat, or the tray it comes on. Similarly, one vegetable is all vegetables. The soupe du jour is the soupe du mois . . . de l'année . . . de l'Éternité . . .

This explains why the patient is invited to order anything he wants from the kitchen. When your order arrives, it will be indistinguishable from what you would have got anyway. You also understand why each meal tray is accompanied by a slip listing the menu items. The menu is the meal's only ID. I learned to make a game of it – guessing what each dish on the tray was by looking at and smelling it, then checking with the menu to see how close I'd come. I consistently flunked the mashed potatoes (Cream of Wheat), but my average improved once I learned to relate the type of container to the probable contents: i.e., the liquid in the plastic cup is likely tea or coffee, even though it tastes more like the beef broth in the bowl. When accompanied by a straw which refuses to penetrate the lid of the receptacle, though the patient can bench-press five hundred pounds, what's inside is apt to be milk. But you can have an identification problem when the meat loaf and the carrot cake are equidistant from the puddle of gravy.

I drew up what I considered to be a typical hospital menu:

CREAM OF WHAT
CHICKEN A LA CLINIC
or
MOOT BALLS
HAS BEANS
POMMES FRIGHT
LEMON ANGEL TORTURE
SOLVENT

The diligent folks on the hospital staff are quite accustomed to removing the tray with the meal untouched. There is no recorded instance of a kitchen worker pausing to ask a patient, "Was everything satisfactory, sir or madam?" Food administration would grind to a halt if it invited criticism. Also, it is virtually impossible to stop the meal tray from arriving at your bedside. Regardless of whether you have your jaw wired shut, are fasting for Lent, are unconscious, dead, or simply already nauseated, neither sleet nor pain nor special order will stop the mealman, or woman, from completing the appointed rounds. Thus the amount of food wasted in a large general hospital would feed most of Ethiopia, with enough left over to fill a doggy bag for the hounds of Hell.

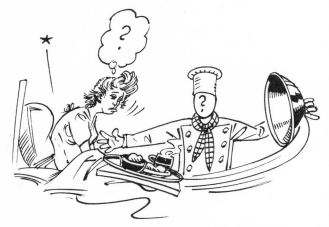

On my first evening, I contributed generously to this profligacy, merely rearranging the swill to avoid hurting the chef's feelings. I considered adding a note: "My compliments to the Chef – the aroma really cleared my sinuses," but thought better of it.

Even had the dinner been related to food, I had

predetermined to eat sparingly, if at all, in order to stall the digestive process. The movement I dreaded even more than Social Credit was the post-op b.m. Reason: surgery is a procedure that gets you on pans and needles. The needles I could tolerate, but I boggled, big-time, at the thought of being put on the bedpan. The steel thundermug. With my back freshly riven? Attempt to mount the shallow crapper unaided? I'd have to be raised and lowered like London's Tower Bridge. Or, worse, helped by a candy-striper, or a male orderly, or a passing group of Little Sisters of the Poor . . . No! No! O constipation, this is thy hour!

I clutched to my breast my doctor's cheerful assurance that I should be able to walk to the bathroom in a matter of hours after the surgery. Walk, crawl, swing on a vine – *somehow* I would attain the face-saving plumbing. Such was my fantasy. I also believed in the Edsel.

A middle-aged, trim woman appeared at the bottom of my bed. "I'm the physiotherapist," she said.

"You're early," I said. "I haven't had the operation yet."

She smiled tersely. "I know. I'm going to show you how to get out of bed."

This promised to be interesting. I have never felt affluent enough to afford a tennis coach, or a flying instructor. Now I was to get a private lesson in something I had been muddling through since crib days: the proper technique for getting out of bed. All I knew for sure about the exercise was that the bed has two sides to get out of – the right side and the wrong side. The latter gives you the grumps for the rest of the day.

"We expect to have you out of bed the day after your surgery," advised the physiotherapist in dulcet Dutch tones. "And valking in your room the next day. Valking in the hall the day after that. Now, please lie on your ztomach."

On my stomach! Gad, here was a novel approach to debedding. She continued:

"Now, pivot on your ztomach so that your legs hang over the side of the bed."

I swivelled on my navel till my undercarriage dropped. No, this definitely wasn't sexy.

"Fairy goot. Now push yourself erect."

I did so. I was now standing facing the bed. "My feet," I pointed out, "are pointed the wrong way. How do I put on my slippers?"

She ignored my question. I sensed that the physiotherapist was on a tight schedule by the way her nostrils were doing isometric exercises. She told me to lie on the bed on my back. "There are a couple of post-surgery exercises you should practise. First, static gluteal contractions – tighten your buttocks."

I suppressed the impulse to tell her that I had been tight-assed since I walked into the hospital. Instead, I dutifully pursed my posterior. Is this how Arnold Schwarzenegger got his start?

"Now, on your side, raise each leg, six times."

You have to concentrate, raising your leg and counting at the same time. Co-ordinating simultaneous physical and mental activities, apart from watching TV and chewing gum at the same time, is not one of my skills. I think it is something that women do better than men, and explains why most physiotherapists are female. And why I was still raising my leg when the physiotherapist walked out.

My next visitor was a tall, blond, insufferably handsome young man who introduced himself as The Resident. As every TV soap-opera fan knows, The Resident is the doctor who never leaves the hospital, even if it is on fire. He is young enough to be still engaged in the learning process, and there isn't a nurse in the building who is not ready, at short notice, to help him complete his study of anatomy.

True to life imitating art, while The Resident was talking to me my room did seem to attract an increased number of nurses eager to take my temperature – gazing at him as the thermometer was inserted in my nose – or check my wristband, or close the window that the previous nurse had opened. Indeed, a whole bevy of nurses entered together, to introduce themselves as the night staff. Whether or not they were disappointed to find me conscious, they were quite decent about glancing at me momentarily, in the presence of the gorgeous medicated hunk towering beside my bed.

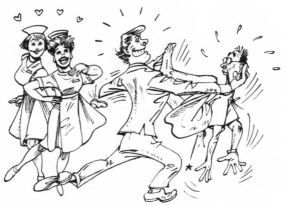

The Resident took my history. Just the highlights. He was more interested in seeing if I could raise my legs ninety degrees, push/pull the palms of his hands with my feet, and resist his dragging my knees apart. It is better to have had these tests than never to have loved at all, but not much. Said The Resident:

"I'll be assisting during your surgery tomorrow."

I was immediately glad that I had not tried to repel his advances. The policy I advise in dealing with people into whose hands you are putting your life is clear:

1) Do not appear immoderately concerned with survival.

2) Flush any assertiveness training down the tube.

3) Fawn as indicated.

"Do you," I asked The Resident, batting my eyelashes, "plan to become a back doctor?"

"No. I hope to do cosmetic surgery."

"Ah!" Should I ask: "While you have me on the table, could you do something about this turkey neck?" No. Risk of overload, comedically. Doctors strive hard to maintain an air of genuine concern for the patient's welfare. If the patient treats his major surgery as low farce, he can hardly complain if the operating surgeon asks the nurse to pass him the slapstick. Some anesthetic gases induce giggles, so it's best to squelch any temptation for the surgical team to lapse into a vaudeville burlesque sketch, hitting one another over the head with a bladder that could be yours. Instead, I said:

"I hope we both have a good sleep." Spoken from the heart. I would have shaken his hand, if he hadn't already left. A nice guy, The Resident. Underpaid, overworked, handicapped by both youth and good looks, he was one of the wonders of our time: a compassionate professional. His parents did a great job with him. Maybe after the operation I'll send them a basket of fruit. . . .

The night nurse brought me a clean hospital gown and undershorts. The gown was blue, the shorts were white, the ensemble enough to break a person's spirit for life. The shorts were new to me and seemed to carry the one-size-fits-nobody principle to the extreme, unless the hospital plans to expand service to include unwell elephants.

Another bizarrerie: the shorts had no fly. Was I the victim of a feminist conspiracy? Or had the shorts been designed by a couturier whose first love was chastity belts? The absence of aperture, front and rear, necessitated the untying of the drawstring and the dropping of the shorts for the most rudimentary of functions. If I, whose interest in clothes is minuscule, found my morale sagging in unison with the seat of the shorts, imagine the effect on a person whose will to live depends on the infrastructure that is his or her lingerie!

To attend to other orifices, I had my earplugs. These also rescued me from the lugubrious sounds from the hospital's powerhouse, which seemed to be located just below my window. Every fifteen seconds the building exhaled a huge, rasping sigh suggesting that the hospital had given up smoking too late and now had chronic emphysema. The only problem with using the earplugs to block out the gargantuan wheezes was that when I woke from sleep I thought I had gone deaf as a result of the surgery. It took me a while to learn to read the nurse's lips. But the life-saving shut-eye more than justified the risk of being the last patient to hear the fire alarm.

There was also the slight chance that I would get my earplugs mixed up with the one for the TV set that hovered blankly above my bed. I don't say that it made much difference to the quality of the dialogue. In fact the only important decision I had to make that first evening in my room – TV, or not TV, that was the question – I postponed till I was sure that I not only had survived the operation but was strong enough to take cable. No way could I succumb peacefully, knowing that I had paid the daily rental fee of $6 for a week in advance.

The blank Cyclops stared down at me accusingly from its swivelly bracket. Odd, when I watch hospital-room scenes on TV I rarely see the set mounted over the bed. Is this because the space-arm monster complicates camera angles? Or do the producers feel that the scene is gut-wrenching enough, without adding the brooding presence of the machine responsible for turning the patient's brain to bat guano?

My mind cleared of this major decision, I lay back for an expected sleepless night thinking about the other threat to my longevity: the morrow's surgery. I was tempted to say a prayer for myself. But since I have been a lifelong agnostic, sceptical of the power of prayer, I had to weigh the efficacy of reinstating a benign God as a one-night stand. I understood better why many writers become born-again Christians after sixty: they want to avoid the embarrassment of pleading with Someone they have continued to argue isn't there. . . .

"Hello, God? This is E. Nicol. I know that I have previously taken the intellectual position that Creation required a primum causum, but that the nature of that cosmic force is unknowable, and to attribute moral qualities to the Creator, let alone the physical appearance of an elderly, white-bearded male wearing a percale sheet, is pathetic superstition. However, if you *are* out there, sir, somewhere in space, and if you *are* both omniscient and not busy right now creating another world and an image that works better than I have, then you know that I feel like a damned fool just mentioning the fact that I am scared shitless, and therefore will deeply appreciate all the help you are unlikely to give me. Amen and awomen."

I clung to my integrity and instead phoned my wife. She said *she* would pray for me. I had never before felt so grateful to have a good, Christian, church-going, God-fearing spouse. I was also glad of the phone beside my bed. It was to prove to be almost as essential to peace of mind as the call-bell nestled under my pillow. Between them they kept me in touch with both the Almighty and the Head Nurse, the Infinite and the Definite. Come what may, I should have no need to call a priest.

"Your surgery has been delayed till this afternoon." My morning nurse lobbed me a smile that I had difficulty returning. I had, as they say in sports, psyched myself up for the matinal rendezvous with Fate. To have Kismet put on hold did nothing for my nerves. Or my stomach. Even though I had resolved to avoid any kind of evacuation except that necessitated by fire or flood, I was hungry. "To hell with your bedpan-phobia," my belly was rumbling. "Send down some grub or I'll order up some liver – yours." To the nurse I said:

"May I have something to eat or drink, retro-actively?"

"Sorry."

Once they write those letters on your chart – N.P.O. – which is Latin for "Don't give this patient a crust of bread or a drop of drink, even if his tongue turns black," you can expect to start seeing the mirages: date-laden palm trees shimmering in desert heat . . . dancing girls frolicking in fountains of vanilla milkshake . . . No matter how long your surgery is delayed, or even if your surgeon has to leave the country suddenly to study a tax shelter in Malaysia, you will continue to live life in the fast lane. You may as well use your fasting to protest something: clear-cutting of forests, abortion on demand, free trade with Mexico. Otherwise it's pointless, lying there with your ribs showing and your little tummy all bloated.

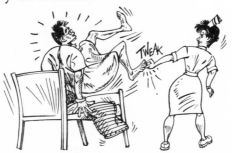

I gathered that I had been bumped in the line-up for the O.R. by emergency cases. Every time I heard the siren of an arriving ambulance, my stomach growled, and I started to worry that if enough people walked into buses and fell in bathtubs, it could be days before I ate again. Such are the imponderables of our overused health-care system. It follows that a patient should not be finicky about the hospital food. Ghastly though it is, eat it up. It may be the last grub you will see for a week, if someone drops a quarter at the Caledonian Games.

I had no chance to get steamed at the delay, as my nurse told me to take a cold shower. Actually she didn't specify cold, but cold was the shower I got, thanks to my usual failure to understand plumbing unless I have lived with it most of my life. For me, shower faucets are like women: I'm baffled as to what turns them on, and chances are I'll get burned. Setting them to project a tolerable blend of hot and cold requires the touch of a master safe-cracker, and I inevitably panic as the shower curtain billows in the storm and the water rises, with no hope of rescue by the Coast Guard. I made a feeble attempt at a disclaimer.

"I had a shower," I told the nurse, "before I left home." This was God's truth. I don't lie about personal hygiene. Too many people may be adversely affected. The nurse was unmoved, saying:

"You have to have a shower *now*. Be sure to wash *everything*, including your hair, with the disinfectant you'll find in the shower room."

The shower room. Sounded pretty damn impersonal. Whatever became of the patient's being tenderly bathed by his shapely, full-lipped nurse? When, and in what nurses' union contract, was the manual lathering of my body replaced by the shower's stark power-wash? Was this another indication of how large institutions like hospitals and universities strive to reduce contact with us, their *raison d'être*? For the college professor, life would be complete if he didn't have to teach students. For hospital staff the goal of improved working conditions is to do away with the patient. Then the teacher could devote himself entirely to research, committee meetings, and sabbaticals, and the hospital worker to study sessions, international conferences, and evaluating colleagues.

Me, the patient, they send to the showers.

Peering out of my door, I confirm that the shower

room lies at the opposite end of the hall. And is occupied (door closed). I see other heads popping out of other patients' doors, all waiting for that shower-room door to open. For some, the distance is a 30-metre sprint. For me, a tough furlong. With hazards like linen carts and patients doddering about in the wrong lane. I'm fairly sure I can overtake the old lady in 508, but the younger guy on crutches could be a problem unless I throw an elbow.

Without warning, the occupant of the shower room emerges. The race is on! And I am beaten by a length – a dark horse from 512. I retreat to my room. After two more futile forays, I force myself to hover outside the shower-room door, my towel over my arm, like a waiter without a table.

Having at last attained the purificatory grotto, I find that I can coax from the faucet only a glacial dribble, fresh off the snow-pack of our local mountains. Determined, however, to be wheeled into the O.R. completely free of torsal fungus and bacteria, I sluice the red disinfectant over my head and body and prepare to scrub myself for the immaculate dissection.

"Open the door!" The voice outside is peremptory. Accompanied by banging. "Open the door!"

"I haven't rinsed," I wail.

"Open the door. Mrs. Williams has immediate surgery. Open up!"

Shit. First my surgery is pre-empted, now my shower. Why didn't Admitting just ask me to take a number? I jam wet feet into slippers, wet body into dressing-gown, wet head into towel, and open the door. The nurse brushes past me, shepherding the wobbly Mrs. Williams. I squish back to my room, disinfected red rivulets streaming down my face, my feet leaving pink puddles. A visitor in the hall stares at me as though I should not be hemorrhaging on the main drag. I spit disinfectant at him and slither into my room. In the washroom I rinse off as much of the sheep dip as I can, but I still smell like something closed down by the city health department.

In this body prep for surgery, I got one break: I didn't need to be shaved. I don't have a hairy back. (I don't have a hairy front either, my chest being just what the doctor ordered for open-heart surgery – though I hope that won't give anyone any ideas.)

For the first time in my life, I was grateful for not being hirsute below the neck. Up to now I had envied the guy with a hairy trunk because it was an assertion of masculinity as well as a way of cutting down heating bills. But one reason why I have kept postponing a hernia operation is that I empathize strongly with the logger who was about to be shaved and said: "Cut all the undergrowth you want, honey, but leave that spar tree standing." I understand that hospitals have largely abandoned the straight-edge razor. I'll need to have that in writing. If I somehow remind the nurse of the wayward husband who cut off her support payments, and she comes into my room holding a leather strop, I'm outa there.

"I'm afraid I can't get my ring off," I confessed to my nurse. My gold signet ring, awarded to me by my parents for having attained twenty-one years of age and thus become eligible to find other accommodation, is permanently lodged behind an arthritic knuckle. It is more a part of me than some of my skin. And I knew, from my previous surgery, that the O.R.

cannot abide jewellery on the patient – wedding bands, earrings, nose studs – under which may lurk flashy germs, ready to swagger into the incision and accessorize my body with a brass-handled box. The nurse looked cross.

"You can't get your ring off?" In her face I read a scorn for sentimental attachment, caused by marriage or finding the ring in a salmon I'd caught. For a moment I thought she was going to order a digitectomy. They remove the finger, pack it in ice, then sew it back on if you need it to write a cheque on discharge.

"I can file the ring off," I told the nurse eagerly, "if you'll bring me a hacksaw."

The nurse shook her head. No hacksaws outside the operating-room? She muttered: "I guess I can tape it." She left to fetch a roll of tape. I had aggravated her workload. I felt rotten. Not for her, for me. There is no way of knowing whether you have been the straw that broke the camel's back till you are up to your navel in dromedary dirt. So, when the nurse returned with the tape and banded my ring, I tried to mollify her.

"Does this mean we're going steady?" I asked.

She didn't appear to hear me. This was the first sign that my voice was not audible to some of the hospital staff. The busier they were, the less audible I became. Maybe the acoustics in my room were bad. But I got the impression that even if I were in Carnegie Hall, vocalizing the request for an extra pillow, they wouldn't have heard me.

In mid-afternoon my wife arrived with spiritual sustenance: a tape recorder and the tape of the John Cleese reading of C. S. Lewis's *Screwtape Letters*. The pre-eminent ex-Python was to prove to be a source of ineffable comfort, in the soul-trying days that lay ahead. *Screwtape* was as close to a religious truss as I cared to get, as a practising agnostic. Though if the operation started going wrong I might have been persuaded to move into something more formally scriptural, namely a complete set of the Holy Bible, the Talmud, the Koran, the Veda, and the Egyptian Book of the Dead.

My wife and I soon ran out of conversation – a situation familiar to relatives attending departures of planes, trains, ships, and gurneys bound for the O.R. For a brief spell my wife even went into the lounge to chat with the kin of other patients who had exhausted all topics of small talk, and compared notes with them about how hard it was to talk with the loved one they were visiting. After all, how many times can you sing, "Will ye no' come back again?" or repeat, "Well, I'm sure everything will work out just fine."

Suddenly the gurney arrives at the door of my room. My wife bids me a cheery farewell, and I'm off, trundled to the elevator that bears me down into the occult bowels of the hospital. I am fully conscious. This alarms me. Surely this is irregular, not to say a serious oversight. Before my previous operation I was given a preliminary needle to make me drowsy, barely aware of what was happening, the arms of Morpheus mercifully clasping me before I even entered the O.R. The question in my mind now is: how far along in the surgery should I let them get before I clear my throat and murmur, "I say, chaps, sorry to interrupt, but I seem to be still awake"?

I am wheeled into the sepulchral gloom of a large circular room with a central bank of electronic gear whose dials glow and blink, a scene I associate with the NORAD command HQ. Someone pushes a button, and whoosh! – I'm off to Baghdad for treatment. . . .

No, the room proves to be a sort of loading–bay, from which the patient can be hustled into one of the adjacent O.R.s without the normal traffic delays. After the stretcher–pusher has parked me on the periphery, I am taken over by the lone nurse in attendance, who is wearing a green gown and a green beret.

Beware the Green Berets! If the candidate for major surgery understands nothing else, he or she should know that joining the company of Green Berets means that the recruit is getting too close to the action. The front lies dead ahead. A matter of one hundred feet, tops. Because of this, the Green Room is where some patients change their mind about having the operation. They leap from their stretchers crying, "Hallelujah! I'm cured – Jimmy Swaggart came through for me!"

The Green Beret checks my wristband and says, "Mr. Nicol?"

This is my last chance. All I have to do is reply, "No, my name is Hassenfeffer. I came into the hospital to deliver some flowers" – and the Universe can resume unfolding as it should. But I lack the courage of my conniptions. I let her take my temperature and blood pressure, which for some strange reason are normal.

"They are just cleaning up the O.R.," says the Green Beret. (*Cleaning up*? Images of hoses and blood-spattered walls.) "They should be ready for you in about twenty minutes." She goes off to greet a new arrival being wheeled in. The only other patient already parked in the room lies flat on his stretcher, eyes closed, body motionless, either unconscious or dead.

Lucky stiff. Is this favouritism? Why can't *I* be utterly out of it? I pay my taxes. . . .

The new arrival, a young guy, asks the Green Beret for a urinal. She draws the curtain around his stretcher and fetches him the vase. I ask for a urinal too. I want everything that's coming to me. Also, among the sources of anxiety vying for my attention is the dread that my bladder will disgrace me in the middle of the operation. Since I shall be lying asleep on my stomach, I assume that I need not fear that other involuntary gaffe, an erection. But my peeing to create a pool table, urgh, it could disgust the entire surgical team, moving them to send me back and order a patient that doesn't leak.

I remember that urinal fondly. It received my farewell tinkle. Not for days would I regain control of the urination that is child's play but a problem for older folks after surgery. For that envoi voiding, however, the sphincters responded loyally, and I was at peace when a tall figure strode into the room and straight to my stretcher. He was Green Beret from head to booties. It was like being approached by a very businesslike Egyptian mummy that had been to med school. Above the mask glinted his glasses, the only sign that this was not The Creature from the Green Lagoon. He spoke through the filter:

"I'm your anesthetist."

"Oh, hi!" – jeez, fancy not recognizing your own anesthetist – "You're wearing a different suit. . . ."

He was already pushing my stretcher towards the swinging doors. Into a corridor flanked by large, closed doors. And, goddammit, I'm still conscious. Surely he's noticed. Don't these guys scrub up everything, including their glasses . . . ?

We hang a left, straight into the glare of the operating-room. Green Berets are moving about, visually unisex, none paying me the slightest attention. No drum roll. No MC announcing, "And now the act you've all been waiting for – Ricky Nicol and His Amazing, Incredibly Buggered Back!". . . .

Whenever I am propelled into an operating-room, I remember Brutus's exhortation to his fellow conspirators: "Let's carve him as a dish fit for the gods. . . ." I'd like to see that message on the wall of the O.R., to offer a smidgeon of reassurance as I am wheeled to the table, where hungry medics brandish their scalpels, impatient to stain their bibs with my gravy, toss scraps of my torso over their shoulders, and set the table on a roar with coarse jokes about my boneless rump.

I was not even received with the cheerful badinage beloved of Hawkeye, of *M.A.S.H.*, Alan Alda relaxing the wounded patient with many a merry quip ("Have you ever had this pain before? Yes? Well, you've got it again. . . ."). Too bad they have to start a war in order to hire good writers for the O.R.

I'm told that soothing music is sometimes played in the O.R., but I've never heard it. Certainly on this occasion I was not invited to select a musical accompaniment from the *carte des ballades*. (My choice would have been the Mormon Tabernacle Choir.) Maybe you have to be in labour. In which case I was lucky to hear nothing. Once, when I was having a root canal, the periodontist asked me whether I would prefer to listen to Bach or Mozart on his expensive stereo system. I said, "Gahh, gahh, gahh." So he played Chopin. I now associate the B-Minor Sonata with being unable to close my mouth.

Bustling. That is the operative word to describe the

O.R. It bustles. Dozens of green people move in different directions without bumping into one another. I sense that they know that I have arrived, or at least that there is *something* under this sheet. From the brisk pace of preparation I realize that the only way today's O.R. can show a profit is by volume. The rapid turnover of patients – onto my face in my case – is vital to keeping the O.R. competitive with the hospital's gift shop or the parkade. I have barely time to admire the décor, the green motif. Everything green is disposable. I pinch my cheeks to avoid matching.

A Green Beret looms over my head. It says: "I'm your surgeon."

My surgeon! "Doctor! Fancy meeting *you* here!" Oh, why, why didn't I get to know him better, when I had the chance? I don't even know whether he's married . . . whether he likes long walks in the rain . . .

Dr. Goodbody gives me a comforting pat on the shoulder. My stretcher is moved closer to and parallel with The Table. I see that it's a surprisingly narrow table. Almost a coffee table. Or an end table. Oh, God, no, not an end table. Please don't let it be an end table. . . .

A huge circular dish of light glowers overhead. It guarantees that a group of complete strangers is going to get a better look at my back than I've had in seventy years of living. I hear the voice of the anesthetist behind my left ear:

"Now, I'm going to give you a little prick on your arm. In a few seconds you will feel a bit weird, then you will sleep."

Good. It's not going to be vivisection after all. Prick. No need to call the Animal Rights League . . . by George I *do* feel weird . . . geronimo! . . .

6

The Wonderful World of Wha' Hoppen?

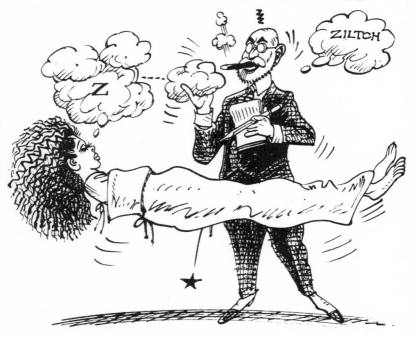

I have had a general anesthetic twice in my life. What I remember most about it is nothing. That is, I have no recollection of the unconscious state. No memorable dreams. Not even a low-grade nightmare. What a waste of subconscious mind! The anesthetic appears to zap the lot – the id, the ego, the superego – the whole can of worms that Freud used to fish for psychosis. The general anesthetic is a mini-death. A preview of ever-lasting oblivion. No wonder it has not caught on as a recreational drug.

No wonder, too, that many people prefer the spinal injection for some surgery. I've never had a spinal. The closest I've come to it has been watching a CBC/TV sitcom. Often my leg goes to sleep after a shot of telly, but I remain awake enough to know that it is time to go to bed. I have to take the word of friends of mine who have had a spinal – for minor operations like the Tupper (transurethral prostatic resection), or hernia repairs – when they swear by the spinal as the best thing since sliced bread. Though of course no one has asked the bread.

Until I had the general anesthetic for back surgery, I was bemused by people who balked at it because they hated to relinquish control of what was happening to them. What the hell, if you're prepared to fly the friendly skies of United, or drink office coffee . . .

This madcap view of the general was changed by my back surgery. For reasons that will become apparent as this chapter struggles to its feet, I now appreciate the positive surgical benefits of biting the bullet. . . .

"What time is it?" I put the question to the person whose face floated hazily above me. I was in the Recovery Room, but had not recovered enough to remember that the Recovery Room was where I would be, if I recovered.

"About eleven. How do you feel?"

"Eleven?" My wits were gathering slowly, like mourners at an economy-class funeral. Eleven o'clock. That meant I had been bye-bye for five or six hours. I once had a stage play on Broadway that had a shorter run than that. . . . I wrote about it in a book with a title that really applies right now – *A Scar Is Born*. . . .

Somehow I was back in Room 502. I don't recall how I got there, but am reasonably sure that I didn't walk it. My eyes focussed on a lanky male nurse standing beside my bed. I couldn't tell from his expression how long he had been standing there, but he didn't need a shave.

"How do you feel?" he asked.

"I'm alive," I croaked. "But that is only a layman's opinion." There was something wrong with my voice. I was quacking like a duck.

"You're alive okay." From his impassive expression I couldn't tell whether he considered this to be an example of medical science working for the good of mankind. "Your wife went home. Dr. Goodbody phoned her to let her know that you came through the operation in good shape."

Why does my wife always get to know something about me before I do? Whatever became of the old-fashioned bedside vigil? Ruined by modern communication, that's what. I'm just lucky that a padre didn't fax me the last rites. I quacked:

"Why are you squeezing my legs?"

"I'm not squeezing your legs," said the male nurse. "The doctor ordered calf compressors for you."

Ah. During his examination of my infrastructure, Dr. Goodbody had murmured something about my veins. He didn't use the word "varicose," but this may have been tact on his part, as he was looking at a pretty fair facsimile of a relief map of Chile.

"The calf compressors help to keep your blood circulating," explained the nurse.

Yes, yes, of course. The older patient, after surgery, is at risk of having his blood use his immobilization as an excuse to stop circulating – something required if the patient is to remain his jolly self – and coagulate. One clot in the bed was enough. A blood clot could wander off to lodge in the brain and leave me prone to seek political office.

The nurse left, and I was alone with my calf compressors. Every ten seconds, by my reckoning, these high-tech garters hissed, constricted my legs briefly, then relaxed their grip. During the several days and nights that I was buckled into the calf compressors I never learned to think of their kneading as a kind of foreplay. Au contraire. Had I not understood that they were clamped to my legs to prevent catastrophe, I would have resented them as being a refinement of the iron boot, an inquisitional torture to force me to confess that the Devil made me do it: abuse my back.

The calf compressors were so novel a device that some of my nurses had never seen one, and when they came into my room were startled to hear the release of compressed air under my bedsheet, accompanied by a billowing of the linen.

"Gas," I told the cleaning-lady. "Don't eat the clam chowder."

To my astonishment, and despite the prosthetic concertinas playing just below my knees, I slept the night after the surgery. My night nurse had to wake me up to ask if I needed a painkiller. (And, yes, they do really wake you in hospital to give you your sleeping-pill.) Declined, with thanks. I was determined to impress the staff – particularly the female staff – as being a tough old turkey. I had heard my wife the RN speak scornfully of patients who demanded Demerol when their suffering consisted of a hurt look. Besides, my back was not paining me that much. It ached some, but I was more concerned that I was still quacking my vocals. It is hard to appear plucky when you sound like Donald Duck.

I slept with three pillows: one under my head, one between my knees – the lower part of my bed becoming quite a crowd scene – and one pillow behind my back. The last served to maintain the designated angle of repose – forty-five degrees. I had been told not to sleep on my stomach or my back, this to "prevent the dressing from oozing." God knows, I didn't want to ooze. Quite aside from getting a nasty memo from the hospital laundry, a person can die of osmosis.

Like the wrestler struggling to keep his shoulders from being pinned to the mat, I lay on my back for no longer than the count of two. I had to give a lot of thought to turning over. Seems like a simple enough project, turning over, unless you are sleeping more than four to a bed. "When Father turns, we all turn," my mother used to say, though I don't remember our family ever slumbering as a combo.

Awkward though the manoeuvre may be, turning over on a hospital bed is essential, if you want to avoid a hip-pointer that would bring tears to the eyes of a Mark Messier. To prevent bedsores, the person considering back surgery should practise turning over in bed with someone sitting on his or her legs. Sleep with a large dog for a month. Or a small pony. Anything to make you strengthen those elbows for the formidable task of revolving the upper body without twisting the back. Watching pizza dough being flipped is not a good role model. Better is to practise rolling over like a log, keeping the knees clamped together and shouting, "Not tonight, Henry!"

Whatever works. You do *not* want to have the fun of back surgery spoiled by your muscles' petrifying because you thought that if you remained immobile long enough, a couple of buxom nurses would rotate you, when in fact they will call in a Finning front-loader. Nurses don't want your bad back. They probably have their own.

"I'm glad to have the back surgery behind me." It was the Morning After, and The Resident had dropped in to scrutinize my dressing. He didn't invite me to look. Nice chap. He even grinned graciously at my pathetic attempt to be jocular though bisected. He confirmed that the operation had taken the better past of four hours.

"With no intermission?" I was awestruck. It had been a long time since I had been able to hold anyone's attention for four hours. It certainly attested to the social value of being a good listener. The Resident said:

"The doctor removed the laminae and large sections of the facet joints at three levels of your spine. Hard work. He showed me the blisters on his hands."

Blisters? *Blisters*? I gave my surgeon *blisters*? I didn't know whether to be ashamed of myself or grateful that they didn't call for a jackhammer. I asked:

"What did you do with my bone meal? I meant to ask you to save it, to put around my roses." I thought it would provide a conversation piece with house guests. "And this is our Peace. I really put my back into grow-ing this rose. . . . "

We were joined by Dr. Goodbody and a young man whom he introduced as a medical student. Displaying no resentment for my back's having blown his plans for the previous evening, as well as mutilating his hands, Dr. Goodbody explained my condition to the neo-phyte surgeon. I, like most other patients, have often been the subject of one of these conducted tours. It gives you the feeling of being a painting hung in a museum – the Mona Loser – while people talk about you as if you were comatose.

The technical exchange between the expert and the student whizzes over my head, and in the student's fixed stare I see nothing to suggest that he will remember me after his final exam. The experience provides a unique insight into being a lab specimen. For this reason some people object to serving as an object lesson in a teaching hospital. But the caring exhibit, like me, finds reward in taking a little of the pressure off the lab monkeys, mice, and rats. Call it an ecological gesture.

I rolled on my side so that the doctor could check my

dressing. He appeared satisfied that the needlework was holding. I asked:

"How long is the incision, doctor?"

"About eight inches."

Eight inches! I have *suitcases* that don't open that far. In none of the back-doctor books had I read of anything larger than a two-inch incision. Two inches is Band-Aid country. A two-inch scar I could cover up with a festive decal – DO NOT OPEN TILL CHRISTMAS. What the books had failed to mention was that the 5 cm slit gave access only for a *discotomy*, the relatively limited decompression of a single disc. Because in my case the nerve was impacted at three different levels of my vertebrae, the surgeon needed to work through more gristle than a roast of the toughest mutton.

With an eight-inch gash, my appearance in a bathing-suit would be flawed. It could put the beach crowd off their fish and chips, and, especially, their hamburgers. I'd have to walk into the surf backwards. Thank God, I never learned to swim.

Shortly after the doctors left my room I discovered a more immediate problem than the blemish on my physique: I couldn't drink. I gagged on the first draft of juice and nearly passed out, fighting for breath. Not only was the juice not getting down my glottis but it was diverting into my windpipe. I wouldn't need to go to the beach to drown. I could do it right here in 502.

This was my first real scare. If I didn't mess my pants then, I could safely assume that defecation was out of the question for the foreseeable future.

When my wife came to visit, I quacked my concern about having to choose between dehydration and suffocation as the way to shuffle off this mortal coil. Good nurse that she is, she at once rounded up The Resident, who peered down my throat.

"Yes, it does look red," he said. He didn't show the degree of consternation I had hoped for. I wanted a shout for Code Blue. If Blue was already taken, by a heart-attack victim, give me a Code Mauve. Puce. Whatever, so long as a trained team of medics scrambled to save my gullet. Hoping to stir The Resident to heroic measures, I said:

"Listen to me try to swallow." I tried to swallow. My throat uttered the dry squeak of the saddle shifting on a camel.

"Your ears wiggled," observed The Resident. A polite attempt to find something noteworthy. Was I overreacting to choking to death?

Half an hour later a nurse wheeled into my room a hanged plastic bag, hooked on its steel gallows. "We're putting you on an IV," she said, and left. Not so much as a by-your-leave, or would I sooner be put on a slow boat to China.

I lay gazing at my new companion. The bag bulged with a clear liquid whose purpose I understood: to induct a glucose solution through the tube into a vein, where it relinquished responsibility. Aside from inoculations and blood tests, this was the first time in my life that I would be given the needle by a bag outside the family. Only later would I learn that many hospitals routinely, after surgery, put the patient on the bottle. Personally, I would have preferred to be breast-fed. But, again, no option.

I assumed that the hospital had calmly found a way to compensate for my being unable to swallow. Presumably this would not be a permanent arrangement. If it was, I would have to find a name for the bottle.

Belatedly it dawned on me that my problem was not the bottle but my swollen gorge. A complication! People *die* of complications. Complications are the most popular way to exit the hospital feet first. Now is the time for the patient to panic. Quietly, mind you, but firmly. Throw a tantrum, but don't hit anyone. Scream pianissimo. Do whatever is necessary to interrupt the smooth transition into condition critical.

The Resident had told me the probable cause of the blocked food-pipe: the endotracheal tube employed to anesthetize me had chafed my throat over the course of a long operation. It figured. I have an unusually narrow pipeline from mouth to belly and all points south. It would not respond amicably to being reamed out by a tube that reminded it of that rotten tongue-depressor the school nurse used to put so far back in my yawp that, on one unforgettable occasion, instead of saying "Ah!" I threw up on her.

So, I submitted meekly to the special nurse who came to connect me to the fellow drip. I was to see quite a lot of these nurses – inevitably dubbed the Ivy League – and admire the skill with which most (not all) of them put me on-stream without having to use a tourniquet, divining-rod or other humiliating gear.

Over the subsequent days and nights I learned these *Rules for Living with an IV*:

1) Unlike other marriages, with an IV there is no such thing as no-fault divorce. The blame is always the patient's – and separation can cost you an arm or a leg.

2) Wedded to your wrist, the IV is a gravity-feed mate. This means that if a gun-wielding robber enters your room and barks, "Stick up your hands!" – you should ask him to reword the question.

3) To prevent its kinking like a garden hose and

consequently cutting off your sprinkler system, the IV tube must be fed down the arm of your hospital gown. Your getting *out* of the gown while your arm is attached to the IV is a trick to faze Houdini. I strongly suspected that there was a hidden camera in my room, shooting scenes that would turn up on a TV show called "America's Funniest Hospital Videos."

4) When you turn in bed, remember to maintain a length of slack. (Experience in fly-fishing is useful, if you can think of yourself as the fly.)

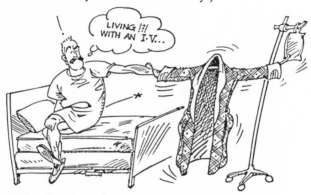

The IV tube may become disconnected at any one of the various junctions along its length, depending on how far you have tried to walk before remembering that you left it behind. Don't leave home without it. If you do, you may see your blood rapidly rising up the tube detached from the bag, the thin red line of heroes from which you would prefer to be excused. When this happened to me, I hit the call-bell with amazing strength, considering that my thumb only works weekends.

The patient is also dependent on the nurse to replace the IV bag when it drains empty, as happens after a few hours. If the nurse forgets this little chore, as mine did more than once, you may brood about becoming dehydrated . . . drip-dried . . . crawling to the nursing-station croaking, "Water! For the love of Allah, water . . . or Pepsi if you have it."

Should the patient complain when a hospital staffer slips up like this? I think not. Unless you are a male patient who (a) is under thirty, (b) bears a striking resemblance to the late Cary Grant, or the early Mel Gibson, and (c) has remembered to remove his wedding-ring, your fault-finding is likely to have the flight pattern of the well-known lead balloon. Remembering that one attracts more flies with honey than with vinegar, I determined early on to be a hive of sycophancy. To be heard muttering about a malpractice suit before you are well clear of the hospital complex invites the rectal thermometer. Inserted with vigour.

7

Look, Doc, I'm Walking!

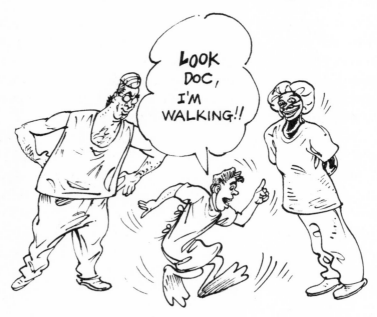

Get the patient out of bed as soon as possible: this is the philosophy of modern hospital care. It doesn't matter whether the patient has had back surgery, a Caesarean, a quadruple bypass, or both legs amputated – the hospital wants you loping up and down the hall in a matter of hours after surgery. It wouldn't surprise me if one day they do away with the beds altogether. A bed just encourages the patient to lie there, when he or she should be ambulant, pickin' 'em up and layin' 'em down, and actively discouraging the body from thinking that what happened was more serious than a razor nick.

Whatever became of those charming scenes in the old British war films where the wounded soldier basked in a Bath chair pushed by a lovely nurse across the languid lawn of a grand estate? When did *convalescence* become a dirty word? Is this the price we pay for socialized medicine, this hustling the patient out of bed and into the Boston Marathon, without so much as a change of shorts?

They had me up on my feet and walking two days after the surgery. I did not walk well. It is said that if it walks like a duck, and quacks like a duck, chances are it is a duck. Well, I trashed *that* theory. I gave fresh meaning to the phrase "faltering steps." But did that dishearten the nurses, the physiotherapist? Not a bit of it. I never saw such a gritty performance as their continuing to make me walk. This despite my spastic gait, as if someone had said to me, "Come to Mummy. . . ."

Even the cleaning-lady seemed anxious to accelerate my mobility. This large Central European person, not given to badinage, trudged into my room with a wet mop which she slopped perfunctorily around the bed, leaving a soapy slick onto which I stepped on one of my first efforts to regain my feet. But for my grasp on the bedrail, I would have slithered to a fast exit worthy of Roger Rabbit. Did I complain? Not on your life, or, more relevant, not on *my* life. But my wife the RN, arriving soon afterward, noted that my socks were soggy. She extracted from me an account of what happened. And despite my croaked protests – "No, no, please, Mary! Don't lodge a complaint, or next time you see me I'll be coiffed with a bucket" – my wife marched off to find the Head Nurse.

Later the Head Nurse swept into my room and made me repeat my description of the accident. I pleaded with her: "No harm done, Excellency. My feet needed the wash. The detergent seems to have soothed my corn. . . . "

Useless. Once the terrible gears of retribution are set in motion, in a large institution, no power on Earth or in Heaven can stay them from grinding to the full length of the shaft. The Head Nurse strode off to her palliative duty of taking a strip off another department.

An hour or so later, the cleaning-lady returned, grim of face, holding her mop in the bayonet-charge position.

"Hi!" I quacked cordially. "Let me guess – first you swab the deck, then you deck the swab – right?"

The cleaning-lady ignored me, peering under the bed, then straightening her substantial body to grunt defensively: "Is *dry*."

"Right on!" Pointless to explain that one look from the Head Nurse had kilned the floor. "Dry as a bone, confirmed by Orthopedics. . . . "

Unplacated, the cleaning-lady gave me a look that said I should be posted SLIPPERY WHEN WET, and she barged away to do battle, a fray whose only casualty would be You Know Who.

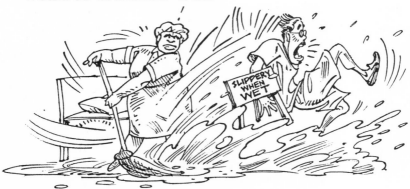

She almost collided with a worker from Food Services who plonked my dinner tray on the buffet beside my bed.

"Thanks," I said, "but I can't swallow."

The worker gave me the fish-eye and backed out. Whether or not I could get the food past my lips was outside her jurisdiction. Her job was to deliver the tray, come hell or high water called soup. I was left alone, a starving man, with an array of smells that my mind, however erroneously, associated with grub.

I mention these contretemps to indicate to the reader how one minor snafu, such as my abraded gorge, can snowball into a situation that would appal Amnesty International. The potential patient has no way of anticipating what mishap will detour the road to recovery onto the Bridge on the River Kwai. True, it may not happen. Some people – you may even have met one or two – have major operations without the surgeon's leaving a sponge in their abdomen, or their rupturing themselves trying to crank their bed up, or their finding broken glass in the rice pudding. But these are flukes. The fact remains, and can hardly be overstated:

You need to be in superb condition to go into the hospital.

Hospital is no place for the sick. You can be in lousy shape and still spend a week in the malaria-ridden, snake-infested jungles of Sumatra without ill effects. But when you surrender your body and, to some extent, your mind to a large, modern medical institution, you dice with Death, mesdames messieurs, unless you are the picture of health, suitably framed.

That is why you ought to get a second opinion before you admit yourself to the hospital. After your own doctor/surgeon has explained why you need to enter the hospital, you should consult a second doctor to obtain his or her professional assurance that you are totally fit, or at least well enough to survive an encounter with today's miracles of medical science. This I failed to do. It was just plain fool luck that I had been taking reasonable care of myself – plenty of sleep, fibrous diet, moderate drinking – the days before I was called into the hospital. Had I been my usual haggard self, I would, I think, be warbling these words to harp accompaniment. All right, Hell's bells.

"You have a bit of a temperature." The night nurse sheathes the digital thermometer whose numbers are all too visible in the dark. "I'll bring you an Aspirin."

"I can't swallow." Maybe I'll get them to print up a sign to post on the wall behind my bed: NOTHING BY MOUTH EXCEPT FRENCH KISS. Yes, I *am* feverish.

The nurse strips off my gown to the waist, slathers rubbing-alcohol on my bare chest, tells me to hold face-cloths soaked in cold water in my armpits, throws the window open to admit the frigid January night air, and goes away. Yes, this should indeed lower my temperature. Odd, though, that such home remedies constitute the cutting edge of fighting fever in today's hospital. What if I had run a temperature in midsummer, when throwing open the window would be contra-indicated? Was I not fortunate to occupy an aging hospital room whose window opened at all? Isn't it expensive, the nurse having to shatter the pane every time a patient comes to the boil?

As I lay there shivering in the dark, arms clasped in refrigerated embrace, I had to wonder again whether this might be the special treatment reserved for the older male patient who reminds the nurse of her stepfather – the bastard who molested her when she was six. With misandry rife in the feminist world, the odds are good that a gaffer like me will be at the mercy of at least one female nurse who sees him as the embodiment of what ruined her life, what is wrong with the world, and what deserves to die before he can do any more harm.

Maybe I should tell the night nurse that I'm gay. My overheated mind rehearses the line . . . "That woman who comes to visit me, she's not really my wife. She's my boyfriend, in drag."

No, it won't fly. A woman can tell when a man is married to a woman. It's something about the eyes – probably the wrinkles. A heterosexual male can't spend a lifetime wincing at photo ads for ladies' lingerie without developing lust lines, horny crow's-feet. I resigned myself to paying the penalty for three million years of male domination.

The night nurse returned, closed the window, took my temperature (unchanged), gave me a recycled cardboard tray to cough my phlegm into, said, "The doctor may order a chest X-ray," and left with the face-cloths, which, I imagined, she would make sure were destroyed as contaminated with Old Boy.

What saved my back bacon was that I didn't have the same nurse for the entire week that I was too fragile to make a run for it. The nurses worked a twelve-hour shift, for three successive days or nights, so that all told, with subs, I had more than a half-dozen women answering my beck and caw. Most of them were too young to have learned to hate men. The very pretty student nurse, who wore a perky cap and a bright smile – as well as the uniform, of course – acted as if no one had yet conditioned her to view caring for male patients as a job for a swineherd.

My *nice* nurses – bless 'em – ran the gamut of the colour spectrum, from coal-black (West Indian) through light chocolate (East Indian) and amber (Filipina) to peaches-and-cream (Newfie). Nothing introduces a person to Canada's multiculturalism more dramatically than being a guest for a week or so at the Waldorf Hysteria. A devout racist could, no doubt, hire a private nurse of a hue to match his bigotry, but I'm too cheap to be a white supremacist.

I welcomed each new nurse that came to my bedside, regardless of race, national origin, religion, or sex – sex being the least negotiable. Nursing is such a dirty, demanding profession that a patient must be grateful that the world still produces so many young women, and a few men, of sufficiently compassionate nature to attend to our various revolting orifices, when they could be more agreeably occupied gutting salmon in a cannery.

However. Today, communication can be a problem.

When a patient is already somewhat disoriented by pain or, as I was, fever, it can be disconcerting to try to communicate with a nurse who *understands* some words of English – "Help!" for instance, or "When is the next bus to town?" – but balks at *speaking* English, for fear of lèse majesté to the Queen's English. Thus it took me a moment to grasp that my nurse's blurting "You dink!" was not a rude remark but an order to take fluid.

I'd wager that in the Tower of Babel the first major crisis was in the infirmary.

Today, the provident and well-prepared patient will try to have some facility in communicating in French, Spanish, Cantonese, and Scottish. I ventured my rusty French to converse with my nurse from Northern Ontario, but it appeared to make her unwell. The rule:

While it would be nice to be able to communicate, never do anything that worsens the condition of the nurse.

Hence I decided not to comment when my night nurse, not knowing her own strength, jerked the pull-ribbon off the light fixture on the wall above my bed. The ribbon – the kind used for Christmas wrap – had been jerry-rigged to the short chain that turned the light on and off and that the prostrate patient could reach only if she or he had arms like an orangutan. To my alarm, the nurse tossed the ribbon in the waste bag.

"*I'll* be glad to tie it back on," I volunteered, gamely raising myself on my elbows. "Just help me up on my knees. . . ."

The nurse shook her head. "I'll have to call the electrician." And she went.

I was left in the inescapable dark. There to ruminate on the tyranny of union jurisdiction. If Flo Nightingale were nursing today, her lamp would have to be carried by a member of the EWU. Forget it that *anyone* could retie that length of ribbon to the abbreviated chain. It would bring the North American labour movement to a grinding halt. An NDP member would rise in the legislature to grill the govenment about patients scabbing in a publicly funded institution. I could be burned in effigy – my best feature.

The electrician arrived a couple of days later. Holsters fully armed with screwdrivers and pliers. Luckily, I had progressed enough to be able to slide on my stomach out of bed before he launched himself at the light fixture, which was working fine, except that it lacked a switch-chain ribbon. He tore the thing apart, replaced the fluorescent tube, ripped out wires, departed to fetch new entrails, returned looking tanned and rested, reassembled the fixture, tested the light, and packed up.

It was not till he had left that I saw that he had not replaced the ribbon on the switch-chain that made the light accessible to me. It was still as unreachable as the sun. I phoned my wife, and on her next visit she brought a red ribbon from our Yule-wrap bin, and she tied it to the light-chain. My wife does not belong to the electricians' union. We took a hell of a chance. But I lucked out – no one noticed the blackleg ribbon. It was still activating the light when I vacated the room. I'd guess that our Christmas ribbon will continue to serve British Columbia's health-care system for years to come. My wife ties a mean knot.

"You leave your dignity at the door," a nurse told me. I found out what she meant on Day Two post-op, when my worst nightmare became reality: Dr. Goodbody ordered that I be catheterized. Despite my desperate pleading, both with him and with my bladder, my miserable micturator refused to yield enough urine to compensate for the intake from the IV. Unless the build-up was relieved, the dammed lake could back up into my kidneys, swell my belly, and eventually necessitate the evacuation of all villagers in the path of the dam's breaking.

Before resorting to the catheter, my doctor did his best to encourage me to void by sheer force of will. "Listen to the sound of running water," he said. So I got my wife to flush my toilet repeatedly while I closed my eyes and imagined that I was nervous about going over Niagara Falls in a barrel. This merely aggravated my catatonic waterworks. So I tuned the TV to watery shows like Jacques Cousteau's scuba-diving . . . *Victory at Sea* . . . No go. The stark fact remained: I was unavoidable.

The reader may not know that there are several types of catheter, none of them the ideal Father's Day present. My wife's nursing manual lists, with illustrations that would be quite comfortable in the pages of *Horror Comics*, no fewer than eight models of this device, for men and women of discrimination. Although I have never discussed it with a woman – the subject rarely comes up at cocktail parties – I gather that for the female, being catheterized is not as traumatic as for the male. For one thing, the physiology is different. Compared to a man's, the woman's route to the bladder is a freeway, whereas his is not built for two-way traffic.

However, the chances are that you – superb specimen that you are – will not need to be catheterized after your back surgery. It is only older guys who develop a drain problem. You will probably get by with a urinal. No, no, not the kind they have in the men's room at the Y. A *portable* urinal. This jolly jug comes in several models, as well as ladies' and gentlemen's urns. Most are plastic, but I was favoured with a heavy pewter flagon that could have been used by Henry VIII to quaff ale. It hooked onto the bed railing, and every time *I* turned – on the hour – the urinal went with me to the opposite rail. A travelling companion, if you will. Visitors may mistakenly put the flowers they have brought you into the urinal, but this should be discouraged, as the blooms may become very aggressive.

Having exhausted the possibilities below my waist, the doctors found a new orifice to penetrate: my nose. My failure to be able to swallow anything but my pride moved them to refer me to the hospital's ear–nose–and–throat man. In none of the scenarios for my back surgery had I anticipated that it would have me rocketing on a gurney to a different wing of the hospital, and into the office of an ENT person, a specialist to whom my sheltered life had never before introduced me. Exciting!

Dr. Entwhistle was a responsive, blue-suited Englishman who listened sympathetically while I quacked my problem up at him as I reclined on my stretcher. He then said:

"Let's have a look at your throat through the 'scope." He fetched forth what looked like a clarinet case, from which he lovingly extracted a length of black tubing with an eyepiece on one end. "Brand new," he enthused, like a violin virtuoso who has finally got his hands on a Strad. I tried to muster equal keenness for the novelty.

Said the ENT doctor: "I'm going to feed the 'scope up your nostril and down the back, to have a good look at your throat. I'll do it very slowly. This 'scope cost five thousand dollars."

I was tempted to wheeze something about paying through the nose, but instead concentrated on receiving a pricey probe that was not to be sneezed at. When he had his vicarious eyeball sited in my post-nasal duct, he peered into the tube and said, "Say 'Eee!' "

I was startled. " 'Eee'?"

" 'Eee.' Say 'Eee!' "

" 'Eee!' " I gave it all I had. I have been told to say "cheese," and of course "ah," but squeaking "Eee!" added a new dimension to the ludicrous. For several minutes Dr. Entwhistle and I eeed at each other, then he retracted the 'scope.

"Yes, your throat is badly swollen," he said cheerfully. "But it should come right in a few days."

I felt vindicated in having complained, yet guilty for having taken the ENT man's valuable time, when God only knows how many patients might be waiting for treatment – to have their Adam's apple wormed, or to remedy an eardrum gone bongo. That night I wakened with a nosebleed, the 'scope having chafed my nostril. I was getting such extensive attention to my post-operative problems that I felt I had to get out of the hospital before it killed me.

I did not mention this concern to my doctors. A trip to the psychiatry department could have been the next step. I shut up, and swore silently that I would be walking in the corridor on schedule (Day Four), unless the hospital paid me to stay out of sight.

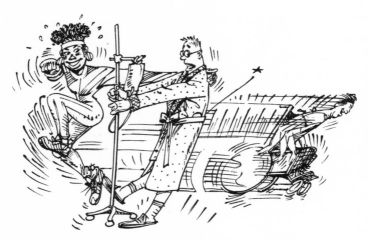

As promised, after the operation the sciatic pain down the legs had been reduced to tolerable. It was my lower back that felt a bit unstable, as though it belonged to someone else, who had failed to take care of himself. My walking motion reminded me of the gait of Frankenstein's monster, when Mr. Peg-neck shucked his ankle clamps and stalked stiff-legged towards freedom. Instead of a bolt of lightning, in my case it was the Dutch physiotherapist who provided the animation.

"Every other step, you must lift your leg high, like zo." She kneed an imaginary groin, making me wince. Since I was still gripping the halberd of my IV, which rolled on devious casters, the total manoeuvre was dodgy, especially when I came on collision course with another back-surgery patient high-stepping down the hall. Our careful, deliberate pacing back and forth resembled slow-motion guard duty by two members of the regiment – The Queen's Own Droopy Drawers.

As a recovering patient, when you start tottering down the hall you have to look out for the young guy in the wheelchair who seems to have learned nothing from his high-speed ramming of a power pole. He lays rubber, accelerating out of his room, passes you on the right (i.e. wrong) side, and jeers when your shaking your fist makes your shorts fall down. The hall should have a pedestrian crossing, but no such luck. Where are the Boy Scouts when we need them?

The hall-traffic hazards worsen during visiting-hours, with the arrival of scores of civilians wearing clothes – God, real shoes! – none of them here to visit you. They wander about the halls, gawking at you as if they've never before seen a person funeral-marching in slippers, with tears streaming down his cheeks. They are often accompanied by their young. The sound of merry little children's laughter is a delight best enjoyed when you can tell them to stuff it.

As for the other patients you meet ambulating in the halls, they represent a cross-section of humanity that you are unlikely to meet socially unless conscripted for war:

• *The Squeaky Wheel.* His call-light is competing with the eternal flame. All his strength has gone to his vocal cords, which can project sound ("Nurse! Hey, nurse!") for distances usually covered only by satellite.

• *The Stoic.* Never complains, or wants to hear you complain. Insufferable. Models behaviour on that of Sioux brave subjected to Sun Dance rites of manhood. Says, "The only way to treat pain is with contempt." Only saving grace is that he has bad breath.

• *The Anal Wag, or Smartass.* Attempts to entertain an entire ward, regardless of size. Has a bottomless fund of stories whose common thread is poor taste. May need to have his bed cranked up till he is folded and packaged for mailing to a hospice for nerds.

• *The Rookie.* Has just been admitted to the hospital. Still has all his own blood, but is clearly nervous. Your gaunt, unshaven face makes his pupils dilate. He or she has many questions about your surgery, which you are prepared, nay eager, to answer, twitching convulsively, and pausing from time to time to ask vaguely, "Did they ever find the *Titanic*?"

• *The Spaced Man.* I was accosted by one of these in the hall, a tough-looking customer who had landed on his head when he fell off a ladder – a stubbled chin, a neck brace, and a brain-damaged attitude. He crossed my T with his wheelchair and, staring at me stonily, growled:

"I guess there's no way outta here."

"I guess not."

"They got us trapped in here."

"That seems to be the situation." (If he rams my IV with his vehicle, I could leak to death.)

"I gotta break outta here. You ready to go over the wall with me?"

"Thanks," I decline, with what I hope is a gracious smile. "I had back surgery a few minutes ago. That drop down the knotted bedsheets to the ground would take a lot out of me. But I wish you all the luck in the world."

He reverses grumpily and zooms off, to scout a more enterprising inmate.

My chances of escape from the institution were enhanced when the nurse disconnected me from my cell-mate: the IV. I was now able to swallow the lemon Jell-O, in such quantity that I shall never willingly eat it again. Since each spoonful took several minutes to slither past my offended larynx, I had ample time to study the seagull. He stood on a window ledge of the hospital building opposite mine, a shabby grey herring-gull, bumming handouts from the occupant of the office within. He was a regular. Always there, a one-bird queue for the food bank. Was this gull forced to accept hospital food because he looked too disreputable to join the other gulls at the garbage dump? Or did the sorry bird represent the wages of socialized medicine? Wouldn't an American herring-gull be out there in the harbour, earning his own scraps by the sweat of his beak? Were we not both dangerously spoiled by the welfare state? (I would later receive the hospital's billing for my rollicking week's accommodation – $4900 – all paid by the province of British Columbia.) Financially, I was as free as the bird. But the sooner I got off that ledge, and once again began foraging for my daily herring, the better. Starting with attention to my post-op exercises.

"Led zee you ride the bike." The physiotherapist had taken me into the floor's gym for my graduation exercises. I had to satisfy her that I could perform the routine before my plea to be discharged from the hospital would reach the higher court – my surgeon. Flunk, and it could be another week of wading through lemon Jell-O, watching that gull sink further into avian squalor. . . .

So, I swung into the saddle with all the alacrity of John Wayne mounting his horse after being shot in the back. "No problem!" I told the physiotherapist, and I pedalled furiously, focussing my mind on winning this leg of the Tour de France and getting to wear the yellow jersey, instead of that grungy hospital gown.

"Fairy goot," congratulated the physiotherapist. "Now you valk up zom stairs."

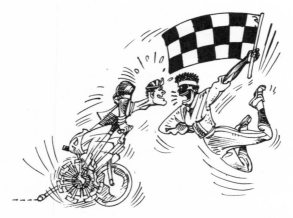

A nurse had warned me about the stairs test. "They won't discharge you till you show them you can walk up a flight of stairs." From that moment I knew how Sir Edmund Hillary felt about climbing Mount Everest. An exhilarating sense of mission. I would have to make the ascent without the Sherpas. The watchers would probably frown on my setting up base camp, or tenting at various levels of the slope to avoid ice storms. They might not even let me use the banister. I had to make the climb to the summit look as effortless as the ascension of Christ, or as using the elevator.

I made it. Not "because it was there," but because *I* was there, and desperate to go home. I did not pause to plant a Canadian flag at the summit, but descended jerkily, displaying no sign of anguish other than knuckles white as the snows of the Himalayas.

"You can leave tomorrow," said Dr. Goodbody. Monday! Exactly a week since admission. I hadn't broken any record for rapidity of recovery from back surgery, but neither was I making my exit in a body bag. Sometimes it pays to be just average.

Maybe I was getting time off for good behaviour. I hoped so. From admission, I had made a strenuous effort to be classified as "a good patient." There is more to being a good patient than refraining from goosing the nurses. It means not being a pain in the ass when the rectum is already stressed out. Easier said than done, because being hospitalized is one of the times that try men's souls, and can make a woman a tad testy too.

The hospital cot is the great leveller. The six-foot-four male executive loses much of his advantage, flat on his back. Itty-bitty old ladies can and usually do show more spunk than macho young men, who statistically have the highest rate of fainting when confronted with a needle. And anxiety will bring forth the selfish streak in a philanthropist, the meanness of jolly good fellows, the courage of a certified wimp, and the patience of an Italian pastry chef.

Assertiveness training may help the out-patient, but once you're in, success depends on the time-honoured strategy of sucking up.

On the Sunday afternoon before discharge I watched on TV an NFL playoff game, knowing that San Francisco quarterback Joe Montana was playing with a bad back. I winced every time he took the hand-off. When he took a hit, I felt it. Little did those feckless young athletes, hurling their bodies through the air with consummate abandon, realize that forty years from now they will be teamed with a back that plays only one position: the huddle.

Shortly after Joe had scored yet another touchdown that will one day cost him his being able to put on his socks without lying on his back, my nurse came to remove my sutures. My last chance to show that I could be blithe in the face of mortal agony. I had of course rehearsed my ad-libs . . .

"It sure has been a fun operation – had me in stitches." Mm, too obvious.

"Hurrah, this is my kind of knit-picking!" Uh-uh. Punning can be harmful to your health in hospital. ("Cut it out" is an expression to avoid there.)

"Be careful which thread you pull – my shorts could fall down." Forget it. These nurses have heard them all. Just shut up, lie on your stomach, and be glad the surgeon used the old-fashioned cross-stitch, instead of the new staples I've heard about. There is something utilitarian about being stapled together, like a mail-order truss, but staples are becoming almost usual nowadays. Staple fare, you might say. Oh, you wouldn't.

In fact I enjoyed the sound of the stitches being snipped, one by one, a homely, domestic scene worthy of Jane Austen. It would have been nicer if we could have done our patchwork beside the cheery fireplace . . . someone at the harpsichord softly playing Purcell. . . .

But at least I didn't seep. Or come unstuck. This had been the last item on my Possible Disaster List: that when they removed the stitches they would find that my wound had failed to bond. A medical first. I would have to spend the rest of my days laced up at the back like an old corset. Afraid to scratch my back lest – ping! I have to pay for a restring. The only advantage would be to make any further operations in the same place a snap. Or a snip.

But the nurse gave no indication that I had come asunder. She coolly taped a large doily over the rift and left me to read the pamphlet the physiotherapist had given me, instructing me in the no-nos and proper exercises to facilitate my return to *homo erectus*. This was all they gave me: a brochure. The doctor had not ordered a back brace for me. There had been no talk of sending a nice hospital bed home with me. Not so much as an alpenstock. I had rather fancied the image of my convalescing on a cane, twirling it for a touch of panache. A cane can be a crutch, of course, but only if you're a midget. Still, I was a bit hurt that they were going to let me walk out of the hospital on my own two totally unsupported feet.

Hospital staff put great faith in the recuperative power of the human body – someone *else's* human body.

While I waited for final clearance, I practised some of the prescribed exercises:

• *The pelvic tilt.* In this mildly obscene exercise, whose alleged purpose is to strengthen tummy and back muscles, you lie on your back on the floor with your knees bent, tighten your buttocks and stomach muscles, and raise your rear end off the floor for a count of five, ten, or ouch-that-hurts. The pelvic tilt is like making love to thin air. It takes a vivid imagination. Without this, you become bored very quickly with the pelvic tilt and start thinking about your income tax.

• *The single leg raise.* "To help limber the back," the single leg raise (on floor) has only one redeeming feature, namely that it is half as difficult as the double leg raise. Unless you are deeply infatuated with your own feet, gazing at each in turn for five seconds can make you wish your body had never bifurcated. You need true grit to stick with the single leg raise for the rest of your life, even with rhythmical accompaniment by the Boston Pops playing "When They Begin the Beguine."

• *Deep knee bending*. This exercise is impossible. For one thing, you have to stand up to do it. Right there it loses my vote for a place in the Top Ten positions. It gets worse. "Stand with your back against the wall." The blindfold is optional. The last cigarette is not, unless you find a wall in the parking-lot. Then, with your head, shoulders, and butt touching the wall, "bend the knees and hold the pose as long as possible. Keep breathing!"

No way. I can bend my knees, or I can breathe. It's a matter of priority. Unless I have been pushed to the rear of a crowded elevator, and for some reason my pants are falling down, I can't muster the adrenaline boost needed to sustain a flawed squat. There has to be an easier way to keep the back limber. Like juggling an elephant with my feet.

But the truly daunting part of your daily ten-minute back exercises is that you must continue to do them for as long as you both shall live. No parole. You may be permitted conjugal visits, or release under mandatory supervision by your cat, but you're a lifer. This back-exercise regime requires an enormous amount of self-discipline – the most boring kind of discipline you can inflict upon yourself. (Unless of course you are already into self-flagellation, leather nighties, ascetic stuff like that. If you can't discipline yourself, give the whip to someone else and tell her/him to get cracking.)

Or, like me, you can do your back exercises while watching TV from the floor. Since there are few ten-minute classics on *Masterpiece Theatre*, I watch children's cartoons at the risk of incurring a herniated mind. Alternatively, you can install a mirror in the ceiling of your bedroom – if you don't already have one, you devil, you – and watch yourself do leg lifts till you lose all respect for the human body.

Some people find that music helps them through their back exercises, though it is not easy to do sit-ups and play the violin at the same time.

8

Score One for Me, Gunga Din

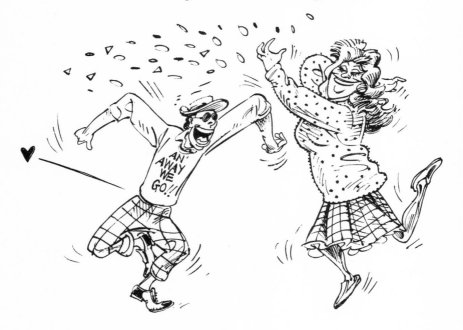

Getting dressed to go home – that I could handle, except, of course, for the adventure with the shoes and socks, and the remote and unattainable feet. In fact, it was sheer, sensuous luxury to sift my body back into a shirt and slacks. Another precious moment was my dumping into the soiled-linen cart the hospital-issue, one-size-fits-nobody underdrawers and the slip-happy gown. I showed restraint, spitting on them only once. I can't speak for women, but for men our manhood depends largely on putting on our pants, almost as much as on taking them off. Younger men, bonded to their jeans as they are, must feel like eunuchs in hospital. Self-esteem is tied to the zipper.

My wife drove me home. It was the first time in a week that I had sat down anywhere but on a commode. Another adventure! Daring, too. The physio brochure had sternly warned against sitting, for several weeks, lest the stitches tear. Bleeding all over the front seat of your spouse's car is not the ideal way to renew the marital relationship. Take the bus, or a cab, if you are chicken about sitting. Another option: *lie down* in the back seat of the family car, and try to ignore the truck drivers gazing down at you with disgust.

The ride home from the hospital is a good time to rediscover the joy of being alive. The grass is greener than green, the sky is bright blue, the birds can fly, look, just by moving their wings! How strange it is, and new – and not an IV bag in sight! You are almost tearfully grateful when your driver stops for a red light. Because you don't want it to end so soon. Nearing

home, you fall in love all over again with the old neighbourhood. Your neighbours – certified creeps before
you went into the hospital – you now see as fellow
human beings. You wave! They don't wave back. No
matter. Wait till their prostate catches up with them.
Especially Mrs. Bagley.

And what a treat, after the tricky business of getting
out of the car and up the steps you'd never really
noticed before, to subside gently onto your own bed!
Getting *off* the bed will be more of a challenge, but
your screams are not going to bother anyone except
members of the immediate family.

And now? Yes, I can now walk, and stand, with less of
that hideous pain down the legs. My verticality is
improved, though still far short of that achieved by
Ubangi women accustomed to carrying pitchers of
water on their heads. At least my hat doesn't fall off.

As for the No. 1 question on the mind of everyone
having back surgery – how long before I can engage in
sex? – it depends, first, on whether you have a private
room in the hospital. Next it depends on whether you
have engaged in sex prior to the operation. Back surgery rarely cures impotence or frigidity, or a sexual
preference for shoes or watermelon. If you were a virgin before your discotomy, chances are you will remain
a virgin for some time after it, particularly if postal
service is reduced further.

Most doctors encourage persons recovering from
back surgery to engage in sexual intercourse in moder-
ation. Tag teams are out. Indeed, you can hurt yourself
just looking at photos of the façade statues on a Hindu
temple. Some of the thirty-two classical positions are

ill-advised, including the ever-popular missionary position, unless the missionary is prepared to accept an abrupt loss of faith. The least potentially damaging posture for the partner of a person recovering from back surgery is the astride, or "ride-a-cock-horse-to-Banbury-Cross," position. Wearing spurs, however, may not be prudent, and exhortative shouts of "Hi-yo, Silver!" are medically off-limits.

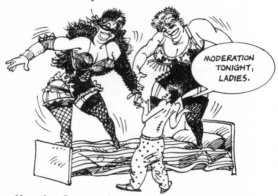

Naturally, before adopting a position on *anything* except distinct–society status for Quebec, the survivor of back surgery will want to discuss it with her/his partner. The "beast with two backs" (Shakespeare) can quickly be reduced to one beast holding a divorce petition, unless both parties agree to the amatory limitations, and find new and exciting ways of just holding hands, playing footsie, and watching anti-erotic videos such as *Nanook of the North*. In most Canadian households, statistics show, the beast with two backs has become the beast with at least one bad back.

Next question: How long before I can go back to work, or stay off work, or never work again? The answer regarding return to your job depends on several factors:

• Were you previously employed?

- Do you have a sedentary job (e.g. auto-racing, tennis-umpiring, pole-sitting)?
- Is your job hazardous to your back (e.g. furniture-mover, logger, unsuccessful political-party leader, exotic dancer)?
- Having spent several recovery weeks mostly lying on the floor, with your feet hooked over a chair, do you now have an irrational fear of heights above three feet?
- Can you lie down on the job (e.g. bed salesperson, psychiatrist, casting director, allied trades)?
- Has your *spouse* gone back to work?

In my case, I was back to work right after I left the hospital. That is the advantage of being a writer who can't afford a word processor and who writes, like Charles Dickens, standing up to a kitchen shelf. But if you intend to return to work that earns you *cash money*, it may be a month or two before you may resume your babysitting, panhandling, ragpicking, etc.

More rewarding than being able to return to work in an upright position, I found, was my gaining stature in the eyes of my wife. "I'm proud of you," Mary told me, "for the way you handled yourself in the hospital."

By God, she was right! I *had* taken on that mammoth institution, and got at least a draw. I don't say that the hospital never laid a glove on me. During various intimate procedures I saw more gloves than you'd find in Eaton's ladies' wear. But I survived, and I might have known, when I saw that the name on the card above my bed was spelled wrong ("Nichol") that the hospital, like any other community of mortals, was not fool-proof. I twigged to that truth in time to take the evasive action that impressed my wife, if not the Hospital Employees Union.

The bottom line – besides the one scarring your lower back – is this: elective surgery does give you a chance to prove that you are a hero or, more likely, a heroine. This is no small achievement, now that our country happily offers fewer opportunities to go to war. Nor can you count on happening to be on a frozen lake at the moment when an inebriated ice fisherman falls into his own hole, affording the chance of heroic rescue. On our streets today, runaway teams of horses are in hopelessly short supply, as are distressed maidens tied to tracks, since the government cut train travel.

You and I may not deserve a medal, for bravery under the command of Major Surgery. But we can rightly take pride in the citation we find in the eyes of a loved one.

Good luck, soldier!

Appendix (Ruptured)

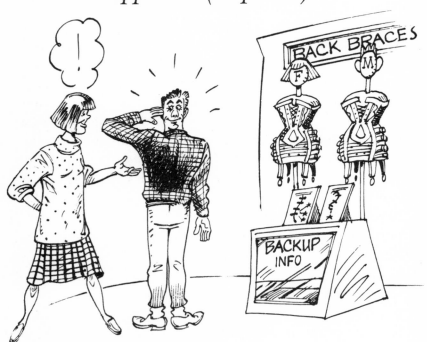

N.B. Like everything in this book, what follows is not serious medical advice, but only the opinion of a layman (sitting or standing is hard for him). Here are some commonly asked questions about the afterglow of back surgery:

Q. You haven't mentioned the chiropractor as a source of relief from post-op back pain. What are you afraid of?

A. My doctor. Some family doctors don't want their patients to see a chiropractor, even from a distance. Without his referral, I would have to *sneak* to a chiropractor, as if I were having an illicit affair. Like wives, doctors have a way of sensing when you are seeing someone else. You have to ask yourself: Is it worth it? On the other hand many people swear by (not at) their chiropractor. It is, they claim, the only person-to-person relationship where you will enjoy being manipulated.

Q. Okay, what about a massage?

A. Love it. But don't get any wrong ideas (wink wink, nudge nudge). Many massage therapists search for pain points in your back by leaning hard with the point of their elbow. They find them.

Q. How about the people who enjoy shiatsu?

A. I don't think diet has much to do with it. And I prefer my seafood cooked.

Q. You haven't said much about *upper*-back problems. Is this class distinction?

A. There is some confusion about where and when the upper back becomes the neck. The vertebrae are of course clearly marked, so that your skull should be able to meet your spine, even in the dark. But it *is* true that cervical spine surgery is more classy than lumbar surgery, because it is less likely to be caused by manual labour. *Note*: this is not *the* cervix. Men have been known to faint, when told that they needed cervical surgery. If in doubt, consult a reputable dictionary.

Q. What about cortisone shots?

A. What about them?

Q. Should I have them to reduce the pain that returns after back surgery and that my doctor says is the result of scarring, which may or may not require another operation? I don't want to become addicted to something that is habit-forming.

A. Damned if I know. But if you feel that way you should keep clear of cigarettes.

Q. Will I be able to play golf after back surgery?

A. If I say, "Yes," you will say, "That's odd – I couldn't play golf *before* my surgery, ha ha." The hell with it.

Q. Get serious.

A. Very well. After back surgery you may walk, walk, walk, ride a bike (especially a stationary bike), walk some more, and go for a nice long hike. Walking in water (not *on* water, which requires special training and bloodlines) is good for you, though it can clear a pool fairly fast. Swimming is always recommended by doctors, though not if you have eaten within two hours (two weeks in the case of hospital food). As for golf and all the other sports people seem to enjoy – hey, you only live once.

Q. My back-doctor book doesn't recommend wearing a back brace after surgery. Did you?

A. Recommend it or wear it?

Q. Wear it, dummy.

A. Only briefly. At one point during recovery I was walking as if my feet had never been formally introduced to the ground. My back felt wobbly enough for me to borrow from my wife the back brace that *she* once wore because of *her* bad back. The back brace resembled a Victorian corset, and although it helped to nip in my waist and define my butt, I found I had to curtsy in order to pick up objects on the floor. This can get a guy thrown out of some pool halls. For a man, the danger in a back brace is not only that it lets the back muscles off the hook but that, after a while, he may start to show an interest in garter-belts. Very quickly a wife's whole lingerie drawer is in peril. Even a woman may be lured into wearing the Merry Widow style of back brace, with dark, textured stockings and spike heels. This can put her into bed before she is ready for vigorous sports.

Q. Yes, um, about that . . . er . . . sort of thing.

A. As I said before – hey, you only live once.

Q. Is it true that bungee-jumping will cure a bad back?

A. Absolutely – expecially if the rope breaks.

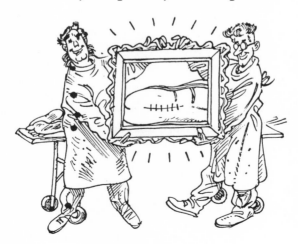

OTHER TITLES FROM

⫿DOUGLAS GIBSON BOOKS⫿

PUBLISHED BY McCLELLAND & STEWART INC.

THE ASTOUNDING LONG-LOST LETTERS OF DICKENS OF THE
MOUNTED *edited by* Eric Nicol
These "letters" from Charles Dickens's son, a Mountie from 1874 to 1886, are "a glorious hoax ... so cleverly crafted, so subtly hilarious." *Vancouver Sun*
Fiction, 4¼ × 7, 296 pages, paperback

AT THE COTTAGE: A Fearless Look at Canada's Summer Obsession *by* Charles
Gordon
"A delightful reminder of why none of us addicted to cottage life will ever give it up."
Hamilton Spectator *Humour, 5⅜ × 8¾, 224 pages, illustrations, trade paperback*

FOR ART'S SAKE: A new novel *by* W.O. Mitchell
A respected art professor and his public-spirited friends decide to liberate great paintings from private collections. When the caper turns serious and the police are on their trail, it's the usual magical Mitchell mixture of tragedy and comedy.
Fiction, 6 × 9, 240 pages, hardcover

OVER FORTY IN BROKEN HILL: Unusual Encounters in the Australian Outback *by* Jack Hodgins
What's a nice Canadian guy doing in the midst of kangaroos, red deserts, sheepshearers, floods and tough Aussie bars? Just writing an unforgettable book, mate.
Travel, 5½ × 8½, 216 pages, trade paperback

WHO HAS SEEN THE WIND *by* W.O. Mitchell *illustrated by* William Kurelek
For the first time since 1947, this well-loved Canadian classic is presented in its full, unexpurgated edition, and is "gorgeously illustrated." *Calgary Herald*
Fiction, 8½ × 10, 320 pages, colour and black-and-white illustrations, hardcover

HUGH MACLENNAN'S BEST: An anthology *selected by* Douglas Gibson
This selection from all of the works of the witty essayist and famous novelist is "wonderful ... It's refreshing to discover again MacLennan's formative influence on our national character." *Edmonton Journal* *Anthology, 6 × 9, 352 pages, hardcover*

PADDLE TO THE AMAZON: The Ultimate 12,000-Mile Canoe Adventure *by* Don Starkell *edited by* Charles Wilkins
"This real-life adventure book ... must be ranked among the classics of the literature of survival." *Montreal Gazette*
Adventure, 4¼ × 7, 320 pages, maps, photos, paperback